Table of Contents

Chapter 1: How the Wolf Method Came to Be

Breathe, it will happen.

"A great adventure is about to begin." – Winnie the Pooh

From the time you were a little girl, did you always dream of being a mom?

I know I did, always.

My family, friends and basically everyone around me always told me that it was my calling in life and I felt like they were right.

As I got to be an adult (like practically every woman today) work and life got in the way.

I started my career in Finance right after going to college at the University of Central Florida.

Go Knights!

I worked like a dog to move up in the company and hey, what do ya know, it worked.

Within 10 years there, I got promoted 4 times and I found myself in a Vice President role.

A few years into those 10 years was when I met my now husband; like me, he was career focused with a growing business of his own.

That focus further pushed back the time that we ultimately decided we would be ready to start our family.

I found myself in my early 30's and now my husband and I were FINALLY ready to pull the trigger, so to speak.

In the back of my mind I worried that we'd be that unlucky couple that struggled with infertility, so I asked my husband to keep our "trying" hush, hush.

Try as he might, he's that guy who just can't contain his excitement (or any secrets in general), so he started telling everyone, "yeah we're going to start trying to have kids in October."

You could practically hear my eyes roll in the back of my head every time this happened, and it happened a lot.

My eye muscles are probably really strong.

So here I found myself, month after month that I wasn't pregnant having to answer the questions about how it was going.

This wasn't so hard at first, but the further and further in we got, the more difficult it became.

Even talking with our closest friends and family about it was really challenging and emotional at times.

Lesson learned, Universe, I'll never ask people how their pregnancy efforts are going again!

It was probably somewhere around 6 months in that the feelings of inadequacy really started to creep in.

What if my husband made the wrong choice marrying me?

He could have been with someone that could pop out babies left and right, but here he is, stuck with old, barren me.

Fast-forward 1 year into trying and I had my first visit to my OBGYN to try to get some insight into why we weren't pregnant.

The best they could do was to prescribe me with the first line of defense for general infertility, before really looking into the route cause.

After a few rounds of a clomiphene citrate (which was supposed to help me ovulate) didn't get me pregnant, it was on to the fertility clinic.

So, after tests, more tests, medications, more medications, emotional breakdowns and more emotional breakdowns, I was basically diagnosed with unexplained infertility with a possible diagnosis of polycystic ovarian syndrome (PCOS).

We were ready to move onto our first fertility treatment of an IUI (Intra Uterine Insemination – basically a fancy turkey baster), but not so fast.

Life threw us a curve ball like no other…my husband was diagnosed with testicular cancer.

This particular type is a young man's cancer, so it wasn't entirely unusual, but still a huge shock.

After a surgery to remove the cancer and one testicle, he was given the okay to monitor rather than do chemotherapy, which was such a relief.

Once he recovered, we were ready to start the IUI process.

IUI 1: not pregnant.

IUI 2: not pregnant.

IUI 3: inseminated on my birthday (has to be lucky), but still not pregnant.

After our 3 unsuccessful tries, we began discussions with our doctor about IVF (In Vitro Fertilization).

It was at this time that my husband started to notice a bit of swelling around his incision site from his surgery.

We went back to the surgeon who suspected it was an abscess and said he'd perform surgery to remove it.

Well, life threw us curveball number 2.

His cancer was back, and this time it seemed much more aggressive.

Since the cancer came back in only 4 months' time (a very rare occurrence for this particular type), his oncologist recommended that he start chemotherapy.

If you don't already know, chemotherapy can completely deplete sperm production.

It's likely temporary, but could possibly be permanent.

So, between both surgeries and before chemo started, we put some semen away into storage and prayed for the best.

Long story short, I'm so happy to say that he's healthy and cancer-free today, but obviously this gave us yet another crazy hurdle to jump over with us trying to start a family.

Talk about an emotional roller coaster.

Thanks to his incredible doctor and team of nurses, after 3 months of chemotherapy was done, his tumor markers were down to a normal number in his blood and scans were all clear!

We then decided it was time to start trying again.

So, with the permission of his oncologist and our fertility doctor, we resumed our efforts of getting pregnant; it was time to start our first attempt at IVF.

We were now met with more and more tests, more and more medications, more and more emotional meltdowns, injections (oh the injections!), and wait, did I mention the injections?

That one round of IVF alone took 7 months from start to finish, but the results were the same.

Still. Not. Pregnant.

Throughout all of those years of me putting the pressure on myself, again what put so much more focus and pressure on it were the people.

Friends, strangers, basically everyone who didn't know we were trying would constantly asking, "So when are you two going to have kids?"

They'd notice that we were married a year, 2 years, 3 years and still no kids.

At some point, instead of realizing that maybe we were dealing with fertility issues (because it's taboo to talk about, right?) they'd start with the, "You have no idea how fulfilling it is to have children. You really should have kids, the clock is ticking!"

As though we didn't want them?

Then there are the people who say, "It'll happen when you least expect it," or "Stop trying and it'll happen for you."

I mean, how is that even possible?

Something you want so bad it HURTS is impossible to forget or ignore.

I kept asking myself, "What is my problem?"

I felt broken.

That's when I decided to take matters into my own hands.

The answer of unexplained infertility wasn't good enough anymore.

So much of what is available on the subject online of trying to conceive is all blog articles and forums.

What kind of real information can you find there?

I'd spent all this time doing what other people told me to do, with no questions asked.

I was a sheep following the herd for no rhyme or reason.

I decided it was my time; time to be a sheep no more.

I am a WOLF.

Okay, fine, yes, it is my last name, but it also represents me taking my journey into my own hands, confidently, aggressively.

This is when what I now lovingly call The Wolf Method was formed.

It was created from my own extensive research, coupled with discussions with doctors of both Western and Eastern medicine and some trial and error.

Conversely, these methods can help to improve male fertility as well, but because women make up the majority of the population that struggle with infertility, I will concentrate on the female aspect.

I found that making slight changes in your daily routine made a huge difference and I wanted to share my findings to get you on the right path sooner than later.

A healthy lifestyle, some vitamins and supplements, coupled with Eastern and Western medicinal practices, but most importantly making sure you are being your own champion, would have you holding your precious little baby before you know it.

I wish I hadn't waited so long to take matters into my own hands.

After 2 ½ years of fertility treatments, I finally decided it was my time to turn things around.

I didn't want to continue on the same path, just following what one person says I should do.

I listened to my body and learned more about my symptoms.

It was shortly after this that I pushed my doctor to do exploratory surgery for possible endometriosis.

She thought it was unnecessary given my current symptoms, but agreed to it because of my husband and I being so persistent.

It turned out that I did have extensive endometriosis.

Of 4 stages, I was diagnosed with advanced stage 3 endometriosis.

I felt vindicated, but somewhat disappointed that this hadn't come up much sooner.

We had 2 ½ years of pain and mental anguish that possibly could have been avoided or at least treated properly sooner.

Now that I had a proper diagnosis, I was finally able to really treat my infertility along with my fertility doctor and my Eastern medicine practitioner.

Change your story; make your time NOW.

YOU hold the key to your fertility.

Chapter 2: The Cycle Diet

Food for Your Thought: What to Eat and When to Eat It to Get Pregnant Now

"May your choices reflect your hopes, not your fears." – Nelson Mandela

You are what you eat, right? In this case, well yeah, it kind of is.

Most women put little to no thought into how what they are eating could greatly affect their fertility.

Well guess what?

IT CAN!

Not only is it important WHAT you put in your body, it's also important WHEN it's put in as well.

Now, I'm not asking for you to completely give up the foods you love.

We all know that the surefire way to sabotage a so-called "diet" (which I assure you this is not) is to completely change the foods you eat on a daily basis to an unrealistic menu.

You definitely won't need to do that.

An easy way to start you off on the right foot, at least in the beginning or throughout if need be, is to make healthy smoothies with nutrient rich fruits.

None of those ice cream smoothies, people, sorry!

Slowly (or quickly) adding these foods to your diet should kick-start you into healthier eating habits.

What I've found that happens along the way is that you start to enjoy eating these foods and your diet naturally becomes cleaner.

Here's an example of some research that was done to prove my case that a nutritious diet and daily habits help to maintain healthy fertility:

A study led by researchers of the Harvard School of Public Health of around 18,000, yes 18,000, women highlighted the significance.

"The key message of this paper is that making the right dietary choices and including the right amount of physical activity in your daily life may make a large difference in your probability of becoming fertile if you are experiencing problems with ovulation," said Walter Willett, senior author and chair of the Harvard School of Public Health Department of Nutrition.

The following are a complete picture of the types of foods you should be consuming at every point of your cycle.

For newbies to the baby making game, your cycle is counted as day 1 being the first day of your period. The cycle of an average woman is 28 days.

Many women have varying cycles, so it's always helpful to track using things like ovulation tracker apps and ovulation testing strips or kits.

These can help you to better identify where you are in your cycle, rather than guestimating.

The following 4 stages of your cycle for the average 28-day cycle are:

Menstruation   Days 1 through 7

Follicular phase   Days 8 through 14

Ovulation   Days 15 through 21

Luteal Phase   Days 22 through 28

I want to note again that the above phases are an approximation of the average woman's cycle and vary from person to person.

Sherri and her husband had been trying to get pregnant for 5 ½ years.

She had spent so much time and money without thinking twice about her diet interfering with their efforts.

After a diagnosis of endometriosis, a failed IUI, and 2 failed IVFs; she decided it was time to make a change.

She switched her diet to whole foods like fresh juices, veggies, fruits and lean meats, cutting out all processed foods.

Within 45 days, she was pregnant!

Here are the foods that should eat and when to eat them to have your own success story during each of those 4 stages for optimal fertility.

What to Eat During Menstruation

- Plant protein (examples are beans, seeds, and nuts)
- Leafy greens
- Beets
- Broccoli
- Cherries
- Raspberries
- Red grapes
- Strawberries
- Citrus
- Meat (limit consumption)
- Fish

This is important because at this time of your cycle, you are likely losing a portion of your stored iron or for those with heavier menstruation, a lot.

These foods will help to replenish those vital nutrients.

Spinach, beans, pumpkin seeds and beets are a great source of iron from plant-based foods.

A great way that I was able to incorporate a lot of these into my diet without flinching was to add spinach or other leafy greens, nuts, and seeds to my daily smoothies.

Trust me, you can't taste the spinach at all!

You can get plenty of iron from a plant-based diet, so make sure to limit your meat consumption.

If and when you do eat meat (in very limited consumption), make sure you're checking if they are treated with steroid hormone drugs or antibiotics.

You want to stay away from those.

Some studies that I've read concluded that there is a link from increased hormones in meats and dairy to ovulatory infertility.

The easiest way to make sure you're avoiding this is to replace the animal proteins with plant proteins.

You'd be surprised at how full you'll feel from eating things like nuts and beans.

Instead of a burger, try a veggie or black bean burger.

You'll save yourself a ton of calories and trust me, they're really yummy.

My husband is a huge meat eater, but after trying black bean and veggie burgers, he was turned.

He'd go searching out the best ones, even asking people on social media for their recommendations and of course he'd already tried them all!

Another way to reduce your exposure to hormones and antibiotics in meat is to buy local or organic.

Now, I know, organic can be expensive, but more and more stores are carrying organic products.

Peoples' eyes are open to the dangers of hormones and antibiotics in their foods and retailers see the growing popularity.

Because of this, there is a lot more competition and prices are trending downward.

In order for livestock to be sold as organic, it has to meet certain criteria:

- They can only be fed vegetarian, organic feed
- They cannot be treated with any antibiotics
- They cannot be treated with hormones

- The meat cannot be treated with radiation
- They are raised in areas that allow access to the outdoors and they can exercise

It's best to get your additional iron from foods, although iron supplements are available.

If you are iron-deficient, then it is best to speak with your doctor before adding in any additional supplements.

Also, remember to get more Vitamin C to help your body absorb that additional iron intake.

Examples of foods rich in Vitamin C are citruses, strawberries, peas, cantaloupe, broccoli, red peppers and tomatoes.

It's also important to note that you'll want to eat sugary and starchy foods in this phase.

Try replacing that cake or cookie with something healthier like some fruit or one of those smoothies.

What to Eat During the Follicular Phase

- Green veggies
- Leafy greens
- Avocados
- Eggs
- Fish
- Shellfish

- Plant proteins (mainly flax)
- Cold-pressed oils
- Whole grains
- Legume

During this phase your body is producing additional estrogen because you are in the process of developing that one ever-important follicle.

One of the goals during the follicular phase is to rebuild a healthy uterine lining from what was shed during menstruation.

Another equally important goal is to support the maturation of a healthy egg.

These foods help your body metabolize the estrogen being produced during this phase.

Beans, especially black beans, have natural occurring estrogens called phytoestrogens.

More black bean burgers, guys!

These foods may even help your body to better manage and get rid of environmental estrogens from foods like dairy and meats.

Foods like avocado, leafy greens, sweet potatoes, olive oil, nuts, and seeds and loaded with Vitamin E.

Vitamin E is found in the fluids of the follicles housing your eggs.

A dish I love and my husband asks for on a weekly basis incorporates a few of the above items and is so quick and easy to make.

It can be an any time of the day dish.

I get a rice and quinoa blend that's microwaveable or you can make it on the stovetop within minutes.

I layer that and some black beans on the bottom of the dish and add some hot sauce and sometimes some salsa.

On top of that I slice up half of an avocado and top it all with an egg, cooked your way of course…my favorite is to cook it over medium.

The yolk gets nice and runny but not too much and makes the dish so rich and decadent tasting.

Ugh, I'm drooling just thinking about it.

Overall, this dish takes maybe a maximum of 10 minutes and is such a hit.

Challenge yourself to come up with quick, creative dishes that incorporate these ingredients without making it too difficult and time consuming.

The second you decide that you're going to put these foods together in the most complicated dish possible is when we slide into old habits.

It's important to slowly become more comfortable with adding these foods if they are not in your everyday diet.

What to Eat During Ovulation

- Plant protein
- Leafy greens
- Fish
- Eggs
- Legumes
- Whole grains
- Cold-pressed oils
- Organic whole milk dairy products
- Plenty of water

This phase is the first half of your dreaded 2 week wait.

Ugh, I know!

Am I pregnant, am I not pregnant?

My boobs are sore, is that from my period coming or a little baby in my belly?

I felt a little twinge, was that implantation?

I'm spotting a little, period or baby?

Well set that mind game aside for a minute and indulge me in the technical side of this part of the Cycle Diet…

For this part of your cycle, your body needs nutrients that will help to release the egg, encourage implantation, promote cell division, and produce progesterone to sustain pregnancy.

Essential fatty acids, zinc, and vitamin B are of the most important, which the above foods are plentiful in.

A lunch or dinner that I like to make is a southwest style salad with mixed, leafy greens (spinach, kale, etc.).

On top I'll add a little bit of whole-fat cheeses like cheddar or pepper jack, black beans, pumpkin seeds, carrots, and just a little bit of a southwest dressing (I know, it's not ideal, but you have to start somewhere and sorry, I want my fatty dressing every once in a while - you have to cheat a little).

Once you get comfortable with a diet that consists of more plant-based foods than animal-based, it becomes a lot easier making it a habit.

You'll even start craving those foods and forget all about the bad ones.

You'll also need to drink plenty of water.

The additional water intake promotes better circulation, which will aid in thinning out the cervical mucous, creating a nicer pathway for fertilization…

…if ya know what I mean (wink, wink).

I like to keep a bottle (my preference is a glass bottle to avoid BPAs) with me throughout the day.

It acts as a reminder to drink water since it's always with me.

If you need it, set a reminder in your phone every hour or less and chug away on command.

Add a few natural flavor drops to your water if it'll help.

What to Eat During the Luteal Phase

- Leafy greens
- Yellow and orange fruits and veggies
- Figs
- Sweet potatoes
- Warm food

This phase falls during the second half of your 2-week wait.

This half is even worse than the first.

More questions, more wondering if this month worked…

Stop it and worry about what you do have control over.

Giving yourself the best chance possible to really feel that pitter patter of a baby inside of you.

You'll need things like beta-carotene to help regulate hormones, which will in turn help to prevent chemical pregnancies (early miscarriages).

Beta-carotene is mostly found in things like carrots, leafy greens, and sweet potatoes.

Bromelain, an enzyme found in foods like pineapple, has been found to help with implantation.

It acts as a blood thinner, pain reliever, anti-coagulant and are anti-inflammatory.

Pineapple is sort of a "superfood" at this stage in baby making, but make sure you're eating it at the right time and in the right quantity.

After ovulation or just prior to IVF embryo transfer, you should consume around one to two half-slices of pineapple each day.

If you eat pineapple during the pre-ovulation phase, it may work against you.

Also, eating too much during this phase (the luteal phase) may work against implantation.

Having more than recommended can cause mild contractions and slight blood thinning.

You should also avoid taking aspirin and eating pineapple in combination, as it may thin the blood too much.

Many women swear by it and eat the flesh as well as the core of the pineapple.

If you do choose to try out the pineapple theory, fresh pineapple is better than canned.

The canning process can deplete a lot of the bromelain.

Alright, enough about pineapples already…they are tasty though.

Another important part of the luteal phase is eating warm foods.

Eating things like soups and stews at this time is important in order to keep your uterus warm.

Cold food and drinks can make blood move to your digestive system, away from your uterus.

So, eating warm foods will create a more ideal environment for supporting pregnancy.

Breaking out the good old slow cooker is a great way to get your warm foods in.

Try being creative and taking foods from your fridge and pantry that seem like they might make a tasty stew or soup.

It's a great way to get rid of things like veggies that may go bad otherwise.

Adding a little vegetable stock and spices to your leftover veggies, beans and leafy greens can make a mighty tasty meal.

Trust me and try it out, it's better than you think!

Chapter 3: The European System

Vitamins and Supplements to Combat Infertility

"You may have to fight a battle more than once to win it."
– Margaret Thatcher

Now, changing your diet is probably one of the best things you can do to kick-start a healthy lifestyle in your pregnancy efforts…

…but the next step is adding in vitamins or supplements that you cannot otherwise easily get from your diet.

Just like with your diet, most women are shocked to find out how much getting these vitamins and supplements into your systen can affect your fertility.

Ideally, making these changes today is important, but having a bit of a lead-time may be even more helpful, especially before you continue any expensive fertility treatments.

It takes your body anywhere from 70 to 90 days to make a mature egg (from the pre-ovulatation to ovulation).

Many of the studies I found all say the same thing.

Your body needs at least 90 days of these changes in order to produce healthier eggs.

I can actually say that I've seen this proven time and time again.

The first time was with my own experience.

I began taking a mixture of additional vitamins and supplements (aside from the prenatal and calcium I was already taking) at the recommendation of my doctor.

The additions were Coenzyme Q10 (better known by CoQ10), DHEA, Omega 3 Fatty Acids, and Vitamin D.

Within less than 60 days of taking my first pill, my second egg retrieval resulted in a 200% improvement in healthy embryos.

It was clear that it had a significant effect on my egg quality.

It's then that I started my real research on vitamins and supplements for fertility.

I shared my experience with Sarah, 31.

She and her partner were trying to conceive for 1 year and 7 months.

They finally decided to move onto fertility treatments, which were also unsuccessful for 6 months.

She decided it was time to add in a few natural remedies of her own to boost her chances before their next try.

She added a prenatal vitamin and Coenzyme Q10 into her regimen and guess what?

2 months later she was pregnant!

Colleen, 42, and her husband were trying to conceive for over 2 years.

She miscarried twice because of poor egg quality, and after speaking with me, she decided it was time to make some changes.

Now, while most women might start slowly, she was sick of wasting time and decided to make a complete shift all at once.

She made a total change in her diet, reduced caffeine, ate more greens, reduced stress, but most importantly added in Coenzyme Q10 and DHEA.

And in just a little over 2 months later, she was pregnant too!

Ok, I know those were a lot of examples, but like I said, I've seen it time and time again.

It really is amazing how effective something you can get from your local drug store really is.

And I do have to give out the generic warning to make sure you always remember to talk to your doctor on proper dosages.

The below are general guidelines, but should never be a substitute for going to your doctor and asking for his or her recommendations first.

Depending on your levels, dosages will be adjusted to better suit your needs.

These are all generally considered safe and super helpful in assisting women to get pregnant and maintain a healthy pregnancy.

At first I had a hard time remembering to take all of the things that I was supposed to.

My prenatal was 3 times a day, omega and calcium twice a day, and vitamin D and CoQ10 were once a day.

I had to take them 6 hours after my thyroid medication which I took right when I woke up.

Then, most needed to be eaten with food, so this balancing act was tough, not only to remember but to space them out properly.

So, since I couldn't be home for every pill, I brought them with me wherever I went in one of those daily pillboxes.

I know they aren't always the most attractive, but they are very useful in kicking this into a habit.

I also had to set reminders on my phone so that I could better space out the timing…and of course be reminded in general to take them.

Taking so many supplements became a bit of a headache and the last thing I wanted to do was feel bad or guilty if I didn't get the outcome I wanted because I didn't take my vitamins right.

I found that it became a habit and I beat my reminders most of the time after only about a couple of weeks.

Folic Acid

This is an absolute must have!

You'll need this to make sure your baby is as healthy as he or she can possibly be.

Before we knew the benefits of adding folic acid to our diets, babies were being born with neural tube defects, which affect the brain and spinal cord.

Taking folic acid has shown a huge reduction in neural tube defects, some say up to a 70% decrease.

Folic acid has been highly recommended for some time now, since we now know how much it helps with issues like these.

It can also help your body to make red blood cells and one study even showed folic acid helped women ovulate.

It looked at women who took multivitamins with folic acid for 6 days a week or greater.

The results were that they had a 40% lower risk of anovulation (lack of ovulation), as compared to women who didn't take the supplement.

Folic acid is also known as vitamin B9, in case your multivitamin or prenatal vitamin has it labeled otherwise.

Some people prefer this vitamin in its natural form, which is called folate (either are fine).

Any doctor you talk to will say that as soon as you are ready to even think about having kids, you should make sure that you are taking a vitamin that includes folic acid.

Like I mentioned before, at the very least you should be taking a supplement with folic acid for at least 3 months before you start trying.

If your family has a history of neural tube defects, or if you have diabetes, a body mass index of over 30, celiac disease or you take epilepsy medication, your doctor may prescribe you higher than the "normal" dosage.

The recommended daily dosage is about 400 mcg.

Coenzyme Q10

I know I mentioned it earlier, but this is more commonly referred to as CoQ10.

It's an antioxidant that does exist naturally in our bodies.

Our cells use it for growth and maintenance, decreasing the damaging effect of free radicals on the reproductive system.

It is needed for basic cell functioning, generating energy in our cells.

Although most studies relating to CoQ10's effect on female fertility are preliminary and ongoing, this supplement has been shown to improve blood flow to the ovaries, with great improvements in egg quality.

It is believed that our levels of CoQ10 that naturally occur in our bodies diminish with age and with the results I've seen, I definitely agree.

I'm about to get even more technical on you guys again, sorry, but I know at least some of you want to get a basic understanding of why this works.

CoQ10 is considered to be the "power source" for the mitochondria, which is where our cells find and use energy.

Having the right amount, or enough of CoQ10 to supply appropriate energy to the mitochondria allows the cells (eggs) to function at their highest capabilities.

This led researchers to believe that if the egg had sufficient energy reserves, that the additional CoQ10 might improve egg quality by reducing chromosomal abnormalities since the eggs would be performing at their highest capabilities.

Makes sense, right?

If that was too technical, I'll put it in layman's terms.

Basically, the older we and our eggs get, the less CoQ10 is naturally found in our bodies.

Our eggs are usually happy and have tons of energy when we're younger, a lot of which is thought to be because we have enough CoQ10...

...but as we start to age our eggs get slow and ornery like we do, or in other words not as healthy.

When we give our bodies the CoQ10 we need, we can re-energize our eggs, making them healthier and happier.

CoQ10 comes in 2 forms, ubiquinone (conventional CoQ10 pills) and ubiquinol.

Ubiquinol is thought to be the more efficient form, since our bodies have to convert ubiquinone to ubiquinol before it can be absorbed.

After the age of 30, our bodies have a harder time converting to ubiquinol, but it doesn't usually have a dramatic effect until later in life, so conventional CoQ10 is usually fine.

I personally didn't take it for my first IVF cycle and that was because my doctor hadn't suspected an egg quality issue, and neither did my husband or I.

Like I mentioned earlier, I started taking it for less than 60 days before my second IVF cycle and I ended up having a significant increase in healthy embryos.

My doctor recommended 600 mg of CoQ10, which is above average, but more than typical may be prescribed if your doctor suspects an egg quality issue.

You can likely consume up to 1,200 mg safely per day, but it's always best to check first with your doctor if you think you aren't getting enough.

The recommended daily dosage for adults is typically 30 to 200 mg.

Omega 3 Fatty Acid

It is true that you can get Omega 3 Fatty Acids through fish and some plant or nut oils, but chances are you probably aren't getting enough of it through your diet alone.

There's no way that our bodies can produce these fatty acids on our own, so adding an Omega 3 supplement to your regimen may be essential in making sure that you are meeting your dietary needs.

It looks like Americans may have the lowest intake of Omega 3s through our diets alone, so we could definitely use the help of a supplement.

I'm probably worse off than most because I don't often eat fish, so this is absolutely necessary for me.

As for fertility issues, Omega 3 Fatty Acids can help you to ovulate more normally, regulate your cycle, increase the flow of blood to the reproductive organs, regulate hormones, and increase cervical mucous.

In recent studies, mice with higher levels of Omega 3 Fatty Acids were shown to produce higher quality eggs.

Increases in Omega 3 Fatty Acids have not only been associated with an increase in egg quality, but also with embryo quality improvement as well.

It is not yet clear how exactly the Omega 3 Fatty Acids help the ovaries produce better quality eggs, but adding this supplement to your daily regimen is shouldn't do you any harm.

Researchers say that the 2 best Omega 3s for fertility and a healthy pregnancy are eicosapentaenoic acid (EPA) and docosahexaenoic acid (DHA).

While DHA is a very important factor in improving fertility and having a healthy pregnancy, DHA depends on EPA to fully function.

Most prenatal vitamins have a healthy amount of DHA in them, but you'll need to make sure that you are also getting the right amount of EPA as well to ensure you are using it to its highest potential.

Recommended daily dosage is 650 mg, of which 300 mg should be DHA and a minimum of 220 mg should be EPA.

Calcium

We all know calcium to be important for tooth and bone health…

…but did you know that it could also help you get pregnant and maintain a healthy pregnancy?

Calcium is fundamental in also helping your baby grow healthy teeth and bones as well as healthy nerves, muscles, and heart.

Not only is it important in fertility and fetal health, but calcium can also help reduce the risks of high blood pressure and preeclampsia while taken during pregnancy.

One particular study also showed that calcium made the reproductive tract more alkaline.

This type of environment seemed to cause the sperm to move their tails in a whipping motion, propelling them towards the egg.

An alkaline environment is also important in follicular development.

It's crazy to think that this supplement that we thought was only good for one or two things is responsible for so many other factors in the creation of our babies.

Just make sure not to overdo it, your total daily intake should not exceed 2,500 mg (and that's in total between both food and supplements).

High levels of calcium can prevent iron absorption, which is very important to avoid, as you will see below that iron is an integral part of maintaining a healthy fertility.

There are some fertility medications that can deplete your calcium reserves, so make sure you are checking with your doctors with any new medications for dosage recommendations.

The recommended dosage is at least 1,000 mg a day (split dosages, as our bodies cannot absorb more than 500 mg at a time).

Iron

Surprisingly, a lot of women may have iron deficiencies and not even know it.

It is thought that low iron levels can be associated with infertility.

Signs of an iron deficiency (also known as anemia) may include fatigue, weakness, chest pain, shortness of breath, cold hands and feet, dizziness, brittle or weak nails, low blood pressure, chronic headaches, and poor appetite.

Anemia is defined as a condition where the body doesn't have enough healthy red blood cells to carry oxygen to your tissues and organs, including the reproductive ones.

This lack of oxygen may cause the eggs in the ovaries to become weakened over time.

It was discovered that women taking iron supplements were at about a 40% lower risk of ovulatory infertility.

This means that, when taking the additional iron supplements, researchers found that those women were able to yield higher quality eggs.

Iron also helps to increase your blood supply, which is vital for conception and pregnancy.

Keep in mind that you can get iron from a lot of different food sources, so supplements may not be necessary.

And like I mentioned earlier, getting iron from supplements isn't ideal, but may be necessary for some.

You should also know that iron toxicity is not normally found from adding iron-rich foods to your diet, however you can overdose from iron supplements.

An overdose from iron supplements can be deadly, so be sure to work with your doctor to see if you have a deficiency before beginning to add iron supplements.

Talk with your doctor before taking iron supplements for proper daily recommended dosages.

Vitamin D

I think by now we all know that we can get adequate amounts of vitamin D from being in the sun.

But the problem is that so many of us are afraid of exposing our skin to the damaging effects of the sun.

There's a real fear of getting skin cancer or, let's be honest with ourselves, we don't want to look older by getting more wrinkles and sun spots from the sun!

It's believed that about 40% of women of reproductive age have a deficiency in vitamin D.

This was one of the first vitamins that my doctor prescribed to me, since I don't get a healthy amount of sun exposure.

Skin pigmentation makes it hard to exactly say how much sun people need get in order to get their daily requirements of vitamin D.

It's said that the darker your skin is, the less likely you are to absorb the UV-B rays, but it also depends on the clothes you are wearing while in the sun along with a few other variables like cloud cover and air pollution.

Someone who is fair-skinned and wearing a tank top and shorts may only need to be in the mid-day sun (time of day is important as well) for 10 minutes a day with no sunscreen.

Someone of Hispanic origin may need 15 to 20 minutes, and darker skinned (African-American or Indian for example) may require 6 times the sun exposure of the fair-skinned person.

Many of us just aren't getting that kind of exposure on a daily basis, so it may be necessary to up your vitamin D through food or supplements.

This vitamin plays a vital role in aiding in the absorption of calcium, zinc, phosphate and magnesium.

Some studies suggest that having the right amount of vitamin D is linked to a higher implantation rate and decreased infertility.

A few studies were conducted with patients undergoing IVF, since it's done in a controlled environment where the entire conception process can be followed.

The studies found that the women with higher levels of vitamin D were significantly more likely to achieve pregnancy compared to women with lower levels.

The daily-recommended dosage of vitamin D is 2,000 to 4,000 IU per day, depending on where your levels currently stand.

See your doctor to find out what the right dosage is for you to achieve an appropriate level of vitamin D in your system.

Zinc

Zinc is in shorter supply in much of our foods today because of poor soil health.

Heating and cooking foods can also reduce the zinc in foods by half of what may have been found in their raw form.

Our lifestyles may also be depleting the zinc that we may be otherwise getting.

Cigarette smoke, pollution, stress and alcohol can all cause zinc depletion.

Making sure you get enough zinc in your diet can be difficult, so if necessary supplements can be taken.

Zinc has been shown to help women use progesterone and estrogen more efficiently and enhances your ability to ovulate.

It has also been shown to help a woman's body produce a healthy, mature egg and can aid in maintaining proper follicular fluid levels so that the egg can safely pass through the fallopian tubes into the uterus.

If you think you aren't getting enough zinc in your diet, talk to your doctor.

Your prenatal supplement may already have enough zinc, so make sure to check before adding a separate supplement to your diet.

Safe recommended dosages may vary between 15 mg and 30 mg, depending on your body's needs.

Chapter 4: The Red-Light Plan

Don't Sabotage Your Hard Work

"Courage is going from failure to failure without ever losing enthusiasm." – Winston Churchill

Now that I've told you about some of what you should be doing to increase fertility, let me tell you some things to avoid.

Every bite you take, every drink you sip is either fighting disease or feeding it.

You're working so hard to make this miracle of a tiny human.

Add into that the emotional stress, financial stress, and physical stress.

You don't want to sabotage all the hard work you are doing to reach this one ever important goal, right?

Let me give you a real-life example.

29-year-old Jennifer was having trouble getting pregnant for 3 years after the birth of her son.

She had no trouble getting pregnant with her son, so she was shocked when time kept ticking away and she still wasn't pregnant.

After nearly a year passed, she decided she was going to take a break from trying and make some lifestyle changes before she would resume trying to have baby number 2.

She was very serious about making these changes not just to try to have a baby, but to feel better too.

She cut down her coffee to one cup a day, completely cut out alcohol, added 3 days of moderate exercise and committed to a healthier diet.

After losing 30 pounds and feeling like a new person, she decided it was time to start trying again.

She was shocked to find out on their first try after these changes that she was pregnant!

"It's amazing how your life can completely change from making changes that were not only better for me, but for my future children," she said.

"I love the way I feel, which makes it so much easier to avoid making the same mistakes that I did. The only thing I'm bummed about is gaining back the weight I just lost," she said with a giggle.

In this next chapter, I'll go over what you can do to further enhance your chances of getting pregnant through some lifestyle changes.

Again, the key is to slowly introduce these habits (or lack-thereof) into your life.

It's so easy to get into bad habits, so I definitely know how hard it is to break them.

In the next sections, I'll show you some easy ways to make these changes that worked for me and so many others...

Limit Caffeine

Stop right there.

I know what you're thinking, "I NEED my coffee, I can't function without it."

Trust me, I really get it…more than you know.

When my doctor told me this I nearly lost my damn mind.

I'd read about it before she told me, but still thought, that's got to be the least of my fertility problems.

I mean, I eat well, I take vitamins and exercise, I can have some vices.

Well, that's partially right.

The recommendation is to limit your caffeine intake to the equivalent of 1 cup of coffee a day (or about 150 mg of caffeine).

For me, substituting another lower caffeinated beverage like some teas and decaffeinated coffees helped me to get through it.

I just needed something warm to start my day and genuinely love the taste of coffee.

It's best to gradually lower your intake so you can avoid major crashes and those terrible headaches from withdrawal.

I know most decaf coffees aren't the most…we'll say, flavorful…but give them a try.

You'd be surprised how much you end up liking them.

I found a brand that offered a decaf (swiss-water method, which is more natural), organic, French roast blend.

It is darker, so not the watered-down tasting decaf coffee you may be used to, and I love it.

So, I don't feel so guilty when I want more than one cup.

Do remember, though, that decaf coffees, teas, soda and chocolate have caffeine in them, so monitor consumption (meaning don't have more than 12 cups, you crazy coffee lady).

I've included average, approximate amounts of caffeine found in what you might be consuming below:

- 8 ounces of brewed coffee – 95 to 200 mg

- 8 ounces of decaffeinated, brewed coffee – 2 to 12 mg
- 1-2 ounce espresso shot – 45 to 75 mg
- 8 ounces of brewed black tea – 14 to 70 mg
- 8 ounces of decaffeinated, brewed black tea – 0 to 12 mg
- 8 ounces of bottled teas – 0 to 40 mg
- 12 ounces of soda (Coca Cola, Pepsi or Dr. Pepper) – 35 to 27 mg
- 12 ounces of Mountain Dew products – 54 to 71 mg
- 8.3 ounces of Red Bull – 80 mg
- 2 ounces of 5 Hour Energy – 215 mg
- 8 ounces of hot chocolate – 2 to 13 mg
- 1.5 ounce piece of milk chocolate – 9 mg
- 1.5 ounce piece of dark chocolate – 31 mg

Recent studies have shown caffeine to have an adverse effect on early pregnancy, with 3 or more caffeinated beverages resulting in an increased risk of early pregnancy loss by up to 74%.

This statistic held true whether the caffeinated beverages were consumed before or after conception.

Another study found that higher consumptions of caffeine daily take longer to get pregnant as compared to women who consumed little to no caffeine.

Caffeine has also been found to inhibit vitamin D receptors.

This limits the amount that is absorbed from the supplement.

Tannins, found in teas (mostly black and some green teas), have been found to bind to iron and block its absorption in the intestines.

If you do choose to drink these teas or caffeinated beverages/foods (again, limit consumption), it is best to wait at least an hour from when you take the supplement.

I know it's hard to switch over, but I did it and I have felt better than I ever did having large dosages of caffeine.

I swore after I cut it out that I may have had a caffeine allergy, that's how much better I felt.

I was never tired and I felt clear headed.

One way to help you get energized without your caffeine fix is if you start your day off with a protein-rich breakfast.

Protein helps you to maintain energy that you otherwise might be losing.

Trust me, if I did it, you can do it too!

Limit Alcohol

Most doctors will recommend that you quit drinking while trying to conceive or at least reduce alcohol consumption.

I mean, of course we know it's better for us to completely cut it out, but if you socialize often, you likely will have a drink or 2 at any particular event, maybe more.

Studies are ongoing and can vary, but overall what seems to be a common theme is that excess alcohol intake can decrease fertility.

Low to moderate consumption of alcohol seems to have little effect on fertility.

So how is "excess alcohol intake" defined exactly?

According to some studies, heavy drinking (on average 5 alcoholic beverages a week or more), has been proven to be associated with increased infertility.

These studies show that consumption of less than 5 alcoholic beverages per week does not greatly reduce your chance of conception.

Here in the United States, a standard drink contains roughly 14 grams of pure alcohol.

So now, you're saying, "aaaand how exactly am I supposed to know when I've had 14 grams of alcohol?"

Well I'm here to help you figure it out; here is a list of what one "standard" drink is:

- 12 ounces of regular beer – about 5% ABV (Alcohol By Volume)
- 8-9 ounces of malt liquor – about 7% ABV
- 5 ounces of table wine – about 12% ABV
- 1.5 ounces shot of distilled spirits (vodka, rum, tequila, gin, whiskey, etc.) – about 40 % ABV

And now at this point you might be asking yourself, "do I drink more than 4 drinks a week?"

You might be surprised to find that the answer might be yes…

…and not because you are ordering that many drinks, but because what you might be considering one drink, may actually be more than that.

We all know that restaurant or bar that is a little heavy handed…and have you actually ever measured out at home what the "standard drink" looks like?

Wine is typically poured somewhere between 6 to 8 ounces and you'll easily get 2 or more shots of liquor in your cocktail.

A couple of glasses of wine with dinner and an after-dinner cocktail may land you in the "heavy" drinking zone before you know it.

So, I think it's no surprise to hear that heavy drinking is associated with impaired liver function.

Your liver plays a role in hormone function, including estrogen and progesterone release.

If your liver is affected by heavier drinking, the disruption to the release of these fertility hormones can clearly affect your ability to get pregnant.

Today, binge drinking and higher alcohol consumption are on the rise.

It may be difficult for some to completely give up drinking, especially in social settings.

For me, a drink in hand meant that people were more likely to stop asking me questions about being pregnant or trying.

I found that discreetly ordering a "mocktail" helped to avoid the hassle and helped to curb the feelings of social pressure.

When I was home, if I felt the want to have a nice relaxing glass of wine at the end of my workday, I got out the wine glass...

…but instead, I filled it with my favorite flavored seltzer water and added a little fruit for an extra added visual appeal.

It felt indulgent just because I was holding stemware that would otherwise be reserved for a nice dinner or special occasion.

Avoid Processed Foods

For a typical shopper, about half of their cart will be filled with processed foods.

You might be thinking, nooo not me, but really observe your cart next time you are in the grocery store.

Canned soups, cereal boxes, frozen dinners, preserved meats (bacon, sausage, jerky), bags of chips, boxes of cookies, candy bars, individually wrapped snacks…need I go on?

Do you shop only on the outer edges of the grocery store where the fresh produce and whole foods are typically found, or do you go down the aisles where the great majority of the processed foods are?

You may be thinking that you are making healthy choices; I know I did, but without even realizing it you may be filling your body with dangerous preservatives and additives.

I mean really think about how long these products can stay on the shelves and in your refrigerator and pantry, what must they have in them to allow that and what are they doing to your insides?

It's simple; our bodies are just unable to digest these extra substances.

Ok, so let me explain (warning: this is about to get technical) …most processed foods contain something called xenoestrogens.

Xenoestrogens mimic the effects of estrogen and are known endocrine disruptors.

When xenoestrogens are introduced to our diets, they can increase the amount of estrogen circulating throughout our bodies.

A build-up of xenoestrogens is associated with infertility, endometriosis and miscarriages.

Additives such as Butylated Hydroxyanisole (BHA) and Butylated Hydroxytoluene (BHT) are also being blamed for infertility and birth defects.

BHA and BHT can be found in foods like bacon, gum, margarine, food coloring, artificial flavoring, canned food and more.

Genetically modified organisms, or GMO foods, are also extremely prevalent in our grocery stores here in the U.S.

GMO is defined as an organism that has had an insertion, deletion, or mutation of genes from other species in order to make the organism more desirable.

This means the modifications in the genetic makeup can help the produce and/or livestock grow bigger, and be insect, drought and disease-resistant.

Studies have found that when animals were fed a GMO diet, infertility, low birth rates, premature births, and higher infant mortality rates resulted.

Additional harmful substances that may be working against you are MSG, sugar, trans fats, and soy.

By doing your due diligence and reading the ingredients on the products you are buying, you can help to reduce your intake.

Generally speaking, the fewer ingredients you see, it is far more likely that you are ingesting less of these nasty things.

I'm a big advocate of organic products, which will fall in line with the less ingredients rule.

Give Up Smoking

Something that may surprise you: both first-hand and second-hand smoke can affect a woman's fertility.

What's most surprising is that passive smoking, or inhaling someone else's smoke, is only slightly less harmful to your fertility than smoking.

Tobacco smoke has hundreds of substances in it, many of which are toxic.

Nicotine and smoking can affect every stage of the reproductive process.

This includes egg maturation, ovulation rates, cervical cancer, hormone production, environment in the uterus, and embryo transport.

Smoking can also increase your risk of miscarriage (the risk increases with the amount being smoked).

10 cigarettes or more a day has been shown to significantly raise infertility rates.

Some studies indicate that smoking can also affect your long-term fertility, even after you've quit.

Smoking can decrease your egg reserve and cigarettes have also been found to cause chromosomal abnormalities in eggs exposed to nicotine.

Once your eggs are compromised, you may not be able to correct the issue.

It's believed that women are born with the eggs that they'll have for the rest of their lives, unlike men who produce new sperm every 3 months.

I don't want this to be all doom and gloom and make it seem like there's no turning back if you're a current or past smoker.

The good news is, once you quit, you can improve fertility within a year of stopping.

If you and your partner both smoke, use each other as a support system to quit together.

Finding a support group, acupuncture, or doing hypnotherapy are all additional options that have great success rates.

Maintain a Healthy Weight

I'm sure you're thinking this section will be about losing weight, but you'd be wrong, well partially anyway.

Having a healthy fertility is dependent on maintaining a healthy weight, avoiding being overweight or underweight.

The best way to gauge this is to check your body mass index, or BMI.

A healthy BMI for fertility is around 20 to 24 (a generally healthy BMI ranges anywhere between 18.5 and 24.9).

You can calculate your BMI by dividing your weight in kilograms by your height in meters…

…or you know, just google it and you can use good old imperial system measurements (feet/inches and pounds) instead and it'll calculate for you.

A BMI between 25 and 29.9 is considered overweight and anything over 30 is considered obese.

Conversely, anything under 18.5 is underweight.

BMI does not necessarily account for the amount of fat versus muscle in your body.

There is some evidence that suggests that the amount of fat in your body plays a role in your fertility.

A body fat percentage of at least 22% is shown to help women regulate their periods.

If you are at a healthy BMI, but you have little to no fat on your body, with more muscle, you may need to gain some fat to regulate your fertility if you are having issues conceiving or have irregular menstruation.

Too little fat can cause a depletion of estrogen.

A lack of estrogen can cause menstruation to cease or be delayed, possibly preventing the body from ovulating.

Underweight women are twice as likely than the average woman to take more than a year getting pregnant.

Planning out your meals for the week can help while adding in full fat dairy items, nutrient dense foods and having 5 meals a day.

Overweight or obese women may also have issues with infertility.

One may be with an increase in insulin.

This causes the ovaries to produce male hormones, which may prevent ovulation.

It has also been found that overweight and obese women have poorer outcomes in fertility treatments.

Ovarian stimulation in overweight women has been shown to produce fewer follicles and fertilization rates are lesser.

Embryo quality is also impaired in younger women who are obese.

A crash diet can be detrimental to correcting your fertility issues.

Gradual, sustained weight loss is beneficial to regularizing your menstrual cycle.

If you have trouble achieving weight loss without crazy diets or other drastic measures, schedule some time with a nutritionist or talk to your doctor.

Work Out a Moderate Amount

So, we all know that working out is a generally healthy activity, right?

It is, but within reason.

Too much or too little can have a negative effect on fertility.

If you forgo physical activity all together and are higher than the BMI listed above, daily exercise can improve fertility.

Too much exercise can cause stress on the body and can be bad for fertility.

It is known to alter hormonal balance, prevent ovulation, throw off the menstrual cycle, and may inhibit conception.

Now, what is considered excessive exercise?

Generally speaking, rigorous, high-intensity workouts are considered excessive.

One particular study showed women who worked out almost every day or until they were exhausted had the highest risk of infertility.

Somewhere around 3 to 4 hours a week of moderate exercise has been found to be ideal.

An example of a good routine would be moderate cardio exercises (brisk walking, dancing, aerobic exercise, swimming, etc.) for 30 minutes a day, 3 to 4 times a week, mixed with 2 days of strength training for 30 minutes per session.

I had a hard time staying in the middle and, to be honest, I still do.

I either want to go all the way, doing an average of an hour work out at least 5 days a week that would be considered rigorous, or I'm just not going to the gym at all.

I found what works best for me is finding a work out buddy or creating a group chat with friends where we motivate each other to get up off of our behinds.

It helps to find something that you truly enjoy doing.

An hour on the treadmill can become very mundane, very quickly.

Trying out alternative workouts like yoga or dance classes can add additional benefits like stress relief while you're getting fit!

Avoid Exposure to Pesticides, BPA, Phthalates, and Other Chemicals

By now, we pretty much fully understand how pesticides, BPAs, phthalates, and other various chemical exposure are dangerous to our health.

Most of us, though, wouldn't think about the effects they may have on our fertility, but they certainly can.

Obviously, it's inevitable that you will be exposed to these at times, but making sure to prepare properly and wear protective gear is necessary.

I think we all pretty much know by now that BPAs are present in a lot of different plastic products.

It's not until you really look at how many products we consume daily that are packaged in plastic that is often not BPA-free that you realize how much we really are exposed to.

You can help limit your exposure by using ceramics, glassware, or non-BPA plastics when heating your foods.

Most plastic water bottles contain BPA, so you should try switching to alternatives such as glassware, porcelain or stainless steel for your water or beverage consumption.

Cut back on canned foods as well, as many are lined with BPA-containing resin.

You can also help limit your exposure by finding packaging that says it's BPA-free when buying canned or plastic encased foods.

BPA is an endocrine disruptor known to mimic estrogen production and can have a negative effect on fertility.

You should also limit your exposure to phthalates.

Phthalates are also endocrine disruptors that are known to have an adverse effect on fertility in women, as exposure can cause implantation failure and miscarriage.

Phthalates can be found in foods like dairy and meat, plastic packaging, toys, detergents, pharmaceuticals, insect repellent, and personal care products like hair spray, shampoo, perfumes, nail polish, and cosmetics.

To avoid phthalates in fragrances, look for labels that include phrases like "phthalate-free" (I know, obviously), "no synthetic fragrance," or "scented only with essential oils."

Plastic products with recycling codes of 1, 2, 4, or 5 should generally be safe from phthalates; however, recycling codes 3 and 7 may contain phthalates or BPA.

Another important factor is to decrease pesticide ingestion.

Phthalates are found in pesticides that are used in conventional farming.

Eating organic produce is an important way to avoid pesticide and phthalate ingestion, as neither is permitted in certified organic produces or pesticide-treated animal feeds.

It is especially important to eat organic when the entire fruit or vegetable (with skin) is being consumed.

Do be wary of labels that claim that they are "natural."

There are no real regulations in the U.S. that would prevent a marketer from claiming something like that.

It doesn't necessarily mean that the product wasn't exposed to pesticides or other harmful substances, so sticking with organic products may be your best bet.

Another chemical that's important to avoid is called perfluorinated chemicals or PFCs.

These chemicals are used in nonstick cookware, breathable and waterproof clothing, and make sofas and carpets resistant to stains, amongst other things.

PFCs are yet another endocrine disruptor.

In this case, studies have shown delayed conception (most ranging in taking over 12 months to get pregnant).

Now, this one may be difficult to avoid in all cases, so beginning by tossing your nonstick cookware and waterproof clothing is a good start.

Another helpful tip would be to remove your shoes when entering your house to avoid brining in harmful pesticides containing PFCs into your home.

Consider Changing Your Skincare and Makeup Products

Okay so here's a fun fact for you:

The average woman uses 12 personal care products per day containing 168 different chemicals in them.

Seriously, check the labels on your products.

Lotions, face washes, serums, toothpaste, and don't even get me started about the number of makeup products I have…

Studies are multiplying that tie infertility to chemicals found in cosmetics and other beauty products.

I said it earlier, and I'm going to say it again, these chemicals, just like so many others we're exposed to every day are typically endocrine disruptors.

Endocrine disruptors can cause abnormal ovarian function and miscarriages.

Some of the chemicals mentioned in the previous section are in your care products, such as parabens, PFCs and phthalates.

We've all heard how many nasty things are in so many products we use daily, but we turn a blind eye to it.

We don't think about how they can affect our bodies.

We're so consumed with the food and medicines we ingest, but we ignore the things that absorb into our skin.

I guess my thought process was always that it's external and it wouldn't really make a difference to my insides, but I was so wrong.

Here's a little idea of some of these chemicals that you can find in your daily care products:

Formaldehyde (used as a preservative in many cosmetics), artificial coloring, behentrimonium chloride (used in most conditioners as a detangler), 2-bromo-2-notropropane-1 (also known as BNPD, 3-diol, or bronopol, onyxide 500, used as an anti-microbial agent in sunscreens, conditioners, and insect repellants), butylated hydroxyanisole (or BHA, one of the top 10 most commonly used preservatives in cosmetics) …

…as fun as listing these wonderful sounding chemicals is (and I could go on for days), you get the point.

In some way, shape, or form, these chemicals have been found unsafe for use in studies and can lead to an increase in infertility.

The best way that you can avoid chemicals like these in your care products are going with organic options.

Grocery stores like Whole Foods often times carry organic and more natural brands that work great and use far fewer ingredients.

The labels often times make sure to mention that they don't use parabens, sulfate, etc.

You can also do a quick Google or app search and download apps or go to websites that are specifically made to provide you with lists of safe products as an alternative.

I made the switch with a lot of the products I use after my first embryo transfer was unsuccessful and I haven't looked back since.

I am positive that the combination of all of my changes with diet, supplements and using more natural products all contributed to my success in the second round of IVF.

Chapter 5: The Breeze Way

Keep Calm and Carry

"We must try not to sink beneath our anguish, but battle on." – JK Rowling

You are what you think.

Sure, your family and friends think they're being helpful with their messages…

…telling you not to stress…

…to stop trying so hard and not think about it…

…but really, honestly, how infuriating is that?

You can't just expect someone to forget about their problems and stop stressing just because you tell them to…

We love them and know that they are trying, they mean well, but they likely are really just adding to your already existing stress.

Sure, you can't put the blame on others for your possible fertility problems, but if you've been taking over 6 months to get pregnant, stress may possibly be a factor.

It's said that about 30% of infertility cases may be pointed back to stress.

Stress can affect a number of things in your body, one of which is fertility.

You could be eating more poorly, drinking more, or smoking because of stress.

Stress on its own can effect ovulation, as well as derail fertilization and implantation.

Let's face it, infertility alone is stressful, procedures are stressful, waiting is stressful.

While we aren't exactly sure what the exact tie is to stress and infertility, it is expected that hormones like cortisol and epinephrine, which are on the rise during times of stress, may have something to do with it.

It is also suspected that a reduction in stress may also increase blood flow to the uterus, which can help with conception.

Some studies found that couples who generally reported feeling good were much more likely to have become pregnant, than those couples who reported feeling tense or anxious.

A large number of infertile couples have not been given a specific cause to their infertility.

This can be somewhat infuriating because how do you know what to fix if you can't tell what needs fixing.

Well surprise, surprise, some doctors believe that in many of the "unexplained infertility" diagnoses that stress is the common factor.

Before I had my true diagnosis, but just some possible causes, nothing concrete, I decided that it was time to cut out as much stress from my life as possible and live my life to the fullest.

I started a moderate workout schedule, which has always been a great source of stress relief for me.

I also started acupuncture (which we'll get into the benefits of in more detail later) and threw in some yoga and meditation.

Jenn, 33, and her husband were trying to get pregnant for nearly 2 years, 6 months of which were with fertility treatments.

Jenn realized that she needed to take a step back from it all and remove some major stressors in her life.

She did weekly acupuncture and after 4 months she found out she was pregnant naturally just before they were set to try IVF!

Theresa, 31, and her husband had been trying for nearly 2 years when they were almost set to start fertility treatments.

The stresses of the pressure from trying to get pregnant for so long was getting to them, so they decided to take some time away from trying.

After a 6-month hiatus, they decided to try again and boom, within the first 2 months they were pregnant!

Some time to concentrate on her wellbeing and their marriage worked wonders for her stressors.

There are many different methods that can work for you to relieve stress and of course, everyone is different.

Of course, if you are facing larger battles and suffer depression or serious stress, these techniques should not replace consulting your doctor or a therapist.

Here are 13 ways that I've found are the most successful in aiding in stress relief.

Get More Sleep

Sleep is a necessity for the human body; I think that's an obvious statement.

It allows our brains and bodies to recharge and rest.

It also helps to repair damaged cells and regulate our hormones.

Some hormones effected by sleep, or lack-thereof, are leptin, progesterone, estrogen, lutenizing hormone (LH), and follicle-stimulating hormone (FSH).

Although researchers do not have direct evidence at this point of a direct correlation to infertility, it is clear that a lack of sleep can cause additional stress on our bodies.

If you are getting less than 8 hours of sleep a night, you might need to pay attention to your routine and make some adjustments.

If you have trouble winding down at the end of the night, start a new routine that you know will relax you.

Taking a hot bath, reading a book, dimming the lights in your bedroom, turning off the television, and putting your phone down are some examples.

Make sure you are avoiding caffeine within at least a few hours of bedtime.

You'd be surprised how long that caffeine can stay in your system.

I had a late lunch with a friend once and had basically a boat sized cup of cappuccino.

I literally felt like I was having a panic attack, the caffeine was getting me so high that I was short of breath.

I couldn't sleep for more than 30 minutes at a time.

I didn't come down from that caffeine high until about 7:00 the next morning and even then I still felt a little jittery.

Everyone's body processes the caffeine differently, so it's hard to pinpoint exactly how many hours before bed that you should cut out the caffeine.

It's safe to say that you know your body and if you're having trouble sleeping and having a mid-afternoon cup, try cutting it out and see if it helps.

Alcohol and cigarettes can also negatively affect your sleep patterns as well, so cutting them out can help.

Alcohol may help you get to sleep, but it's been proven to interrupt your sleep throughout the night.

If you nap during the day, consider stopping if your sleep isn't consistent.

If you try all of these things and you are still having issues sleeping, consider seeing a sleep expert.

Have Sex…for Fun

I know, novel idea, right?

If you're like anyone who has been trying for 6 months or more, you know that having sex starts to feel like a chore rather than the fun it used to be.

Peeing on sticks to see if you're ovulating and timing your sex can certainly add stress to something that should be fun and relieve stress.

Sex releases endorphins and other hormones that improve your mood.

Cortisol is released in times of stress.

It can inhibit luteinizing hormone releasing hormones (LHRH), which in effect cause lowered luteinizing hormone (LH) levels.

If you've done any reading about ovulation or used those sticks I talked about earlier, then you've probably heard of LH and that it triggers ovulation.

Cortisol can also disrupt follicle stimulating hormones (FSH), estrogen, and progesterone.

Overall, these things can create an environment not suitable for fertilization and implantation.

So, have more sex (even when you're not ovulating), reduce cortisol levels, and get those endorphin levels going!

Write It Down

Writing can be a great source of stress relief.

Keeping a diary and being open and honest in it about what's going on in your life can help in many ways.

I know years ago, I got my husband a journal for him to write in when he began to, what I call, loop.

Meaning his head would spin and spin around this one thing (usually business related for him) until he would drive himself crazy and think of nothing else, even after felt that he had some sort of solution.

So, he began using this journal in those moments, which were interrupting his sleep at that time, and the second it was tangible and out of his mind, he was able to calm his mind and therefore his body as well.

Several research studies have been done to support this claim.

One of which was done by Dr. James W. Pennebaker, who chaired the psychology department at the University of Texas, Austin at the time of the study.

He asked 46 healthy college students to write about either trivial topics or traumatic events for 15 minutes a day for 4 days in a row.

For 6 months following his study, the students who wrote about traumatic events were less likely to visit the campus health center and used less pain relievers that the students who wrote about the trivial topics.

Most outcomes of studies done on writing to reduce stress have shown reductions in blood pressure and heart rate.

Initially, writing about personal things may initially upset you, but eventually it is shown to help you relax.

Challenge yourself to try it at least few times before giving up on it and see how you feel.

Take Time for Yourself

Now, this one could mean a lot of different things to any one of you reading this.

To me, it's quiet time taking a bath, cooking, reading a book, or just watching television…honestly I could go on, but these are a nice and simple start.

For my husband, it's hanging out with his friends or exploring any number of his new hobbies he's decided to take up.

Your "me time" may be getting a massage, taking a trip, exercising, meditating, or knitting, it's anything you want it to be.

But in the end, it should be something that you get personal fulfillment and enjoyment out of.

Whichever way you slice it, we all need some time for ourselves to get away from everyday life and forget about things for a while.

With work, social obligations, doctor appointments, caring for family or friends, and/or maybe fertility treatments, we all deserve to do something good for ourselves.

Once we get into the ruts in our daily schedules, it's hard to do something for ourselves.

Before stress from my job and all of the fertility treatments, I would take time to cook and that was one source of stress relief for me.

After a while, I let that go because it just took up more time than I was willing to give with the all of the time that was being taken away by the other stressors in my life.

Eventually, I told myself that I deserved that "me time".

One of the most relaxing nights was when I combined all of my "me time" activities.

I poured myself a nice glass of wine (again, in moderation it's fine), cooked my favorite meal (parmesan and fontina risotto with mushrooms and chicken), ate it (guilt free because cheat meals are ok, again, in moderation), and took a candle lit bath while reading a book.

I felt so relaxed, had an amazing night of sleep, and felt so incredibly rejuvenated and ready to rule the world the next day.

Oh yeah, and an important note to make on this one, put your phones and social media away.

Take this time to really concentrate on YOU and what makes you HAPPY instead of feeling jealous looking at photos of Dan's trip to Monaco or Katie's Hawaiian trip.

Make a list of your favorite things to do for YOU.

Schedule your "me time" on the calendar, I'd suggest once a week if you can swing it or at the very least, once a month.

I find that when something is clearly on the calendar, you will usually hold yourself accountable and complete whatever that thing may be.

In this case, it's something to help you be your best self.

Take Time for Your Partner

Time for ourselves is one of the most important things you can do for yourself, but let's not forget that there is another very important person who is likely feeling a lot of the stress and anguish with you…

…your spouse, partner, significant other, future baby's daddy/second mama.

Sometimes we forget about the importance of a healthy relationship through all of the stress that comes with trying to make a baby.

My husband and I were not immune to this.

A year of infertility and cancer can weigh on any healthy relationship, and it definitely did on ours.

It was hard for me to feel like I wasn't alone, even with him at my side through all of the major events in the fertility struggles.

He was the rock through my breakdowns and reassured me time and time again that he will always be here, that I am not broken, that we're in it for the long haul together.

But even after hearing all of that, it still didn't completely make my feelings of solitude and inadequacy go away.

It took me a while to really hear this, but after my husband's bout with cancer and our subsequent resurgence into the infertility battle, I finally listened to those who told me not to stop living my life, our life.

I avoided so many places and doing so many things because I was so afraid.

Afraid of Zika, afraid of getting shots to travel to certain places, afraid going into social settings for fear of being asked the dreaded questions, fear of allowing us to enjoy our life.

I decided to let go.

I decided I had to continue to live my life, for us.

I needed to let go of all of my paranoias so that we could maintain a healthy relationship.

After that point, we decided now was the time to travel to as many places as we could afford, visit friends, see sites we'd always dreamt of because pretty soon, we'd have a baby that wouldn't allow us such privileges as often or easily.

I know "letting go" is easier said than done, but remember your partner is probably stressing right there along with you, so helping to lessen their load will take so much weight off of both of your shoulders, trust me.

It may take some time for you to get to that point, and that is understandable.

Being open with others about your struggles makes it easier to let go of your fears that will hold you back.

And speaking honestly about not wanting to talk about it is okay too.

Putting yourself in other peoples' shoes is a helpful exercise to remember that it's hard to know how to be around people with fertility issues.

If they haven't dealt with the struggles, they will never fully understand how you are feeling, so letting them know that it's hard to talk about helps.

Pointing them in the direction of articles that explain how it feels to be asked questions that make you uncomfortable when dealing with infertility helps as well.

I was told about a podcast that goes through nearly everything that I'd been through, generally speaking.

Telling my friends and family to listen was a great way for me to share what my experience were like with them without actually having to directly talk about it, which was difficult for me.

Things like this can lessen your feelings of discomfort in social settings, allowing you and your partner to get back to more normal social activities.

Another important part of any relationship is really taking devoted time out for each other.

My husband and I have a weekly date night on Wednesday nights.

It is reserved for just him and I, no double dates and no phones or other distractions.

It could be a simple dinner made at home where we sit at our dining room table, rather in front of our usual spot on the couches in front of our TV, or it could be an activity like a cooking class or rock climbing.

Bringing yourselves out of your usual activities and out of your comfort zones is a good way to shake up to what could otherwise become a mundane routine.

Surprise one another.

Take turns planning these outings, it adds a little excitement and spice into the mix.

That extra spice will also help your sex schedule turn back into the feeling of when you were first together.

This will allow you to go back to the having sex for fun.

I know at a certain point, that could feel forced for some, especially if you've been trying for a long while.

But trust me, adding in some different activities into your schedule will make you feel like you're starting to date all over again.

You'll remember why your relationship was so much fun and exciting all over again.

Exercise

It's no surprise that a lot of people use exercise as a form of stress relief.

I'm definitely one of them.

It helps to produce endorphins, the feel-good hormones, which naturally help to curb your stress.

You may think that you have no time to exercise, but it doesn't take much.

Pretty much any type of exercise or movement can work as a stress reliever, whether it be aerobic, yoga, climbing stairs, or swimming.

Start slow if you haven't worked out in a while.

Building up your fitness level slowly is important, firstly to avoid injuries and secondly to ease yourself into your new habit.

You know that calendar we talked about penciling your "me time" into?

Well use it here too, heck, make this your "me time".

Give yourself credit for doing a good job if all you can do at first is walking up the stairs daily at work.

Take three 10-minute walks throughout a day if you can't fit in one 30-minute session.

Make sure you try to build momentum and set new and higher goals for yourself each workout or each week.

Something that really helps me keep a routine is finding a friend or loved one to work out with.

My husband and I have made it a habit to go to the gym several days a week together.

That motivation pushed us both to create this habit, so when one of us can't make it, the other still goes, which further motivates the both of us.

Remember, moderate exercise is good for your fertility and stress reduction, but excessive exercise could work against you.

The ideal amount of exercise for stress reduction as well as fertility boosting is around 3-4 hours of moderate exercise a week.

Practice Yoga

Yoga has been a long-known process to clear our minds and reduce stress throughout our bodies.

Now I know what some of you are thinking, "Oh here we go, she's getting all Zen and granola on us."

I really was so uncomfortable at my first yoga class, my first 10, but I reached a point in my life where I was willing to commit to anything to reduce the stress I was feeling.

After some time, I was really able to feel the effects of doing yoga semi-consistently (at most once a week, at least once every couple of months).

I'm generally not one to shy away from trying a new workout routine, so this was a good fit for me, but it may not with you.

In a national survey, over 85% of people who practiced yoga reported that it helped them relieve stress.

Yoga differs from other workout routines in that it concentrates on the connection of mind and body.

The belief is that stress resides in either the body or the mind, and that many of us either live in our mind or our body.

So, for instance, my job in Finance lead me to spend a lot of time in my mind, leaving much tension built up in my body.

I know this is true, because every time I've ever had a massage, the masseuse told me how much tension I stored in my neck and shoulders.

In particularly stressful times at work, I'd notice my shoulders raising toward my ears, increasing this tension.

If you do a lot of physical labor or are an athlete, yoga may help you to become more aware of your mental state.

Whichever you fall under, yoga should bring your mind or body to a new state of relaxation, both of which will help with stress relief.

Yoga is a great form of exercise that you can do for small bouts of time (10 minutes, let's say) or spend hours perfecting your poses, so it's a great way to take small breaks in your day or introduce slowly to your morning or after work routine.

There are so many great videos online that you can follow, but typically there are also very affordable classes wherever you may be (my area has a great studio that offers $5 classes).

Try Meditation

Meditation is probably the easiest way to accomplish stress relief, from a time conservation perspective.

You can do it anywhere, anytime, for however long you can or need to.

It can be as formal or informal as you'd like it to be.

Just like yoga, there are plenty of guided options online for you to choose from as a starter.

Yoga studios also often offer classes on meditation (yoga is also considered a form of meditation).

Meditation requires a few basic elements: focused attention, a quiet setting (if you can block out what's around you then that works too), a comfortable position, relaxed breathing, and an open mind.

Be aware of what your body is doing throughout.

Are your shoulders tense?

Relax them while still paying attention to your breathing.

Another thing that many people do throughout their meditations is repeating a mantra.

Whether it is spiritual, religious, or just something that makes you feel good, a mantra can help to clear your mind of clutter and stressful thoughts.

An example of this is maybe a prayer or something like the well-known, "om," or something like "I change my thoughts, I change my world."

It can help to keep your mind focused on that one thing, blocking out all other distractions, allowing your mind and body to become more relaxed.

Don't be too hard on yourself if you feel that you aren't "doing it right."

Meditation is a learned skill and takes some time to perfect, just remember the goal is for stress relief, there's no one way to do it right.

Use Positive Language

We all know that we are our own worst critics.

I'm guilty of this, something goes wrong and I can think of a list of things that I did wrong that may have caused it.

My transfer didn't take on IVF try number 1; of course, it's my fault.

I shouldn't have had that extra glass of wine a month ago, I pushed a shopping cart and held shopping bags after my transfer, but my instruction sheet said not to, I shouldn't have been walking around so much, maybe that's why the embryo didn't take.

I could go on like that forever at times, especially when the stakes were so high.

This is still a work in progress for me, but I strive to "think" better every day.

For instance, instead of saying, "I'm a failure at trying to get pregnant."

Instead, I'd say, "I'm doing everything I can to get pregnant."

Our perception can alter our reality.

Negative self-talk can make you perceive things as more stressful.

For instance, when my cousin was little (probably 3 or 4 – I am 21 years older than her), we went to Disney World.

We took her on pretty much every ride you could imagine there, including Peter Pan and Pirates of the Caribbean.

Now, you'd have to assume that the more likely of the 2 she would be scared during would be Pirates of the Caribbean, but never Peter Pan.

Well the exact opposite happened and I'll tell you why.

The person who rode Pirates of the Caribbean with her made light of the cannons blasting and the dark rooms and she laughed throughout.

On the other hand, person number 2, who shall remain nameless, who rode with her during Peter Pan exclaimed, "it's scary, close your eyes" as they rode through the scene where they're flying above the city streets.

She was terrified, Peter Pan was her least favorite ride, but she LOVED Pirates of the Caribbean.

This is a very primitive example, but one that holds true.

Whether someone is saying it to us, or we say it to ourselves, the power of suggestion and our words are so strong.

Negative talk can turn into a self-fulfilled prophecy.

I become far more empowered when I try to turn my thoughts into positive versions of the same previous negative thoughts.

My husband is great at this; he is his biggest fan (I come in at a close second).

After his cancer diagnosis, he had no doubts he'd be fine, and he was, he is.

His positive thinking allowed him to cope better than most might in that time of stress.

Positive thinking is not only known to reduce stress, but has also been shown to lower rates of depression and increase life span.

At the very least, you can try to be your biggest ally instead of your worst enemy.

What could it hurt?

Chapter 6: The Eastern System

East Meets West: How Traditional Chinese Medicine Can Compliment Western Methods

"It always seems impossible until it's done." – Nelson Mandela

We can learn a lot from our neighbors in the East.

While the idea of traditional Chinese medicine (TCM) may seem intimidating, it may also possibly intrigue you.

I know I've always had some level of curiosity about it.

Either way, it is something you should consider thinking about as a supplement to your current baby making efforts.

For thousands of years, Eastern medicine has been used to treat all sorts of medical conditions in a very different way than typical Western cultures currently do.

TCM believes that the body's vital energy circulates through channels called meridians.

These meridians are believed to have branches that connect to organs and bodily functions.

The aim is to keep the body in complete balance through your physical, mental, spiritual, and emotional health.

Western medicine typically treats the symptom or single complaint rather than the underlying issue as a whole.

For instance, Western medicine might look at irregular menstruation and prescribe birth control pills, while Eastern medicine might try to figure out why the periods are irregular and treat the underlying cause.

TCM will take into account things like your diet, life stressors, or any other number of things that they believe might have something to do with the condition causing that symptom.

Using methods such as acupuncture, herbal remedies, diet, exercise, massage, and foot soaks are common practice.

Many fertility clinics work very closely with TCM practitioners, pairing East and West together to optimize results.

Before I had begun trying, a friend recommended it as it had worked wonders for her.

She miscarried twice, and then had trouble conceiving.

She turned to acupuncture and after about 3 months of treatment, the rest was history.

She now has 2 beautiful children.

She always tells anyone trying to conceive how much it helped her to carry 2 healthy, full-term pregnancies.

I personally was a little apprehensive at first about turning to TCM practices.

As a Westerner, I've been brought up to look at our Eastern counter parts' medicinal practices as "different."

And, well, it is from what we practice, but we can learn something from combining the two.

They balance each other well, where one leaves off, the other picks up.

Overall, these TCM remedies are known to help boost fertility rates through ovulation and menstrual regulation, enhanced blood flow to the uterus, stress relief, and much more.

Studies have been shown to increase the effectiveness (higher pregnancy rates) of Western treatments such as IUI and IVF, when paired with TCM treatments.

TCM is considered a cheaper method than what traditional Western medicine can offer for fertility treatments, from an out of pocket expense (when not covered by insurance).

Most states do not require insurance plans to cover fertility treatments and the ones that do are typically limited.

With mine, for instance, my insurance covered only so much of my medication, so by the time we were at round 2, we were basically out of pocket entirely.

This brought our costs to about $10,000 just for that round alone.

TCM is also generally considered to be very safe with little to no side effects.

I did not experience any adverse side effects, just a little bruising from the acupuncture needles here and there.

If anything, I felt extremely relaxed immediately after and then subsequently revived and had more energy than ever in the days to follow.

If you do decide to try out the Eastern route, give it a real go.

To really experience the full benefits, it is best to visit your TCM practitioner for at least once a week for a month, but optimal amount of time is 3 months.

Trust me, you won't regret at least giving it a try.

Acupuncture

Acupuncture is by far the most popular and widely used form of TCM to treat infertility.

It can be tracked back at least 2,500 years as part of the health care system in China.

So needless to say, the fact that it's still around and being extensively used all over the world says a lot.

Tiny needles going into your skin may be a scary thought to most, but if you find someone who truly knows what they are doing, you shouldn't feel a thing.

Well, maybe a little, but no more than a tap or maybe a tiny pinch on your skin just for the moment that they are inserting the needles, but it should be painless after as you lay on the bed and relax.

With someone who knows what they are doing, side effects should be minimum if any at all (soreness and bruising are among the more common).

Choosing a practitioner that's right for you is important.

Your fertility treatment center or friends' recommendations are a great place to start.

Research the facilities that you are considering; do they provide their credentials and training background?

Most states in the U.S. require non-physician acupuncturists to pass an exam from the National

Certification Commission for Acupuncture and Oriental Medicine (NCCAOM).

You can search for practitioners in your area that are licensed by the NCCAOM on their website, http://www.nccaom.org.

Some insurance covers treatments; so, check your insurance plan before deciding on a facility as well for some cost savings.

If your insurance doesn't cover treatment, but you are still worried about cost, there are community acupuncture centers that are a fraction of the cost of others.

The only downside is that you are in a room with several others being treated, but everyone is usually very respectful and quiet so you can relax all the same.

It's a great option that I know several friends have tried.

Once you've narrowed down your options, the next step is meeting with your acupuncturist.

Talk to them about your diagnoses (if you have any yet) or any symptoms you may have, aside from just letting them know you are trying to get pregnant.

They need as much information as possible in order to provide the right treatment plan.

Your first meeting will likely entail them doing an initial consultation to check a few basic things including your pulse, the color of your face, and the shape, color and coating of your tongue.

That first diagnostic meeting and treatment may take around an hour with the treatments that follow taking about 30 to 45 minutes per session.

Your acupuncturist may ask to see you once or twice a week.

Ideally, they'd like to see you for 3 months prior to any fertility treatments for optimal effectiveness, or if you are impatient like me (at the very least) 1 month prior to treatments.

In theory, acupuncture is used to balance the flow of energy that is moved through the meridians that I mentioned before.

The idea is that Qi (pronounced "chee") is the form of energy that must flow through the body at all times.

When it doesn't, illnesses such as those associated with infertility can arise.

Acupuncture is used to restore that flow and helps to resolve the issues causing the illnesses.

From a Western medicine point of view, acupuncture helps your body to release endorphins, which can help reduce stress and plays a role in regulating menstruation.

It has also been shown to be as effective as drugs like clomiphene citrate in egg production, for those that either can't take the drug or want to try using an alternative method first.

Acupuncture is also known to enhance blood flow, which can help with the uterine lining (aiding implantation) and also helps the ovaries produce more follicles.

It is often used to supplement fertility treatments and has been shown to have higher success rates (in both pregnancies and live birth rates), as compared to those that just do Western fertility treatments like IVF alone.

Herbal Remedies

Often times, TCM herbal remedies are paired with acupuncture to treat causes of infertility.

They can be used as a stand-alone treatment or in combination with other TCM remedies.

If you are taking any prescription medicines, you should first consult with your doctor(s) to make sure that herbal remedies won't affect the efficacy of your medications.

The unknowns of what are in your herbal concoctions might be a bit intimidating or worrisome.

Since the FDA typically does not regulate them, many doctors will recommend staying away from them.

Herbal treatments are generally considered safe, but there is an important way that you can help protect yourself if you are unsure.

A good standard is the same for the acupuncturists, look for someone who is a member of the National Certification Commission for Acupuncture and Oriental Medicine (NCCAOM).

Often times, acupuncture is sufficient on its own if you are younger and have no real diagnosis as to why you aren't getting pregnant.

Conversely, if you are older and have specific issues like polycystic ovarian syndrome (PCOS) or low ovarian reserves for instance, then acupuncture with the addition Chinese herbs will be most beneficial.

Your acupuncturist is will possibly suggest treating you with both acupuncture and herbal remedies, but remember you have a choice.

If the TCM practitioner you choose tries to push you into something that you are not comfortable with, then you are not going to the right one.

This is your body, and as I mentioned earlier, be sure that you are acting as your own champion and that you are fully satisfied with your treatment plan.

Foot Soaks & Warm Feet

I think we can all agree that a nice, warm foot soak and some warm feet sound oh so relaxing.

I personally love my baths, and while they're generally frowned upon during certain parts of fertility treatments, a great alternative is a foot soak.

If you are a person who generally is cold or has cold hands or feet all the time, then this one is especially for you.

In TCM, the meridians for your reproductive organs are all believed to travel to our feet.

Cold feet represent a cold womb.

A cold womb (or cold uterus) basically means you are lacking circulation in that area; this controls ovulation and implantation.

Symptoms of a cold uterus are cold hands and feet, spotting before your period, clots during menstruation, menstrual cramps that feel better with heat, poor libido, repeated miscarriages, infertility, anovulation, lower back pains, low basal body temperature, and/or hypothyroidism.

I don't know about you, but this list was about 90% me.

Although a hot foot soak can help with ovulation, it is most important around implantation (just after ovulation, during your 2-week wait).

I figured, how easy is it to do a foot soak and wear slippers or socks to keep my feet warm?

You can choose to either soak your feet in solely water or with different mixtures of fertility boosting oils or herbs.

My TCM practitioner had packets of herbal mixtures that looked like tea bags that were used to help boost my fertility even more than just warming my feet alone.

Whether you do what I did or create your own special fertility concoction, the general instructions are to bring a pot of water to a boil, place your herbal mixture in the water and bring to a simmer.

Steep your herbal mixtures in the hot water for about 30 minutes.

After that, the water should be brought to temperatures ranging between 100 degrees and 113 degrees Fahrenheit (about 38 to 45 degrees Celsius).

Once you've achieved this optimal temperature, it's time to start soaking.

Leave your feet in the bath for about 30 minutes or to a maximum of 45 minutes.

If the bath cools below 100 degrees Fahrenheit, you can remove your feet and add more hot water until the temperature is back up.

Make sure your feet aren't in the bath at the time so that you don't scald yourself while adding much hotter water to bring the temperature up.

Not only are hot foot soaks important, but also eating warm foods and keeping your feet warm is just as important.

When you aren't doing the foot soak, wear comfy slippers or socks, especially if you live in colder climates.

I personally live in a hot climate, but I have tile floors and we like to keep the air temperature inside lower.

So, walking on the tile without slippers or thick socks can quickly turn my feet into icicles.

Another way to warm your womb is in eating warm and/or spicy foods.

Staying away from iced coffees, cold cereals, and salads during this time in your cycle could do you a world of good.

This is probably the easiest and most cost-effective way to help boost your fertility!

Low Level Laser Therapy (LLLT)

My TCM practitioner introduced me to low level laser therapy (LLLT), or cold laser therapy.

It's being more widely used in Japan and has been studied both there and in Denmark.

Some of these studies are surrounding women considered to be "severely infertile" (average age nearing 40 and have been trying to conceive for nearly 10 years).

The studies showed great success from this form of therapy, even in low doses.

It's painless and from everything that I've experienced myself and read, completely symptom free.

Women have found success using this therapy as a stand-alone or when paired with other assisted reproductive technologies (ART).

LLLT has been shown to help with egg quality, improved circulation, softened scar tissue (possibly from endometriosis), and a reduction in inflammation.

When our eggs are developing, they require a remarkable amount of energy.

As we age, the mitochondria (mentioned earlier in the CoQ10 section - how our cells are energized) begins to wear down.

The mitochondria of older eggs produce much less adenosine triphosphate (ATP), from which the energy is provided to the cells.

LLLT has been shown to increase ATP levels in cells, improving egg quality.

Western medicine has long maintained that this sort of thing is impossible, but as this technology is more widely used, it seems to be combating this stigma.

For something that is painless and without side effects, it's definitely worth a shot!

Chapter 7: The DIY Plan

Before You Call the Doctor

"Parenting begins the moment you make any conscious effort to care for your own health in preparation for enhancing your child's conception." – Carista Luminare-Rosen

Don't pick up that phone just yet.

From a Western medicine standpoint, there are some things that you can do to help your chances of getting pregnant before deciding to go to a fertility specialist.

Many women start with fertility tracking apps and I do agree that they are a helpful tool.

They are a simple and good way to start, but the thing is, they aren't fool proof.

They may be throwing you off when you are timing intercourse if you aren't ovulating when the tracker estimates that you are.

Several friends started using these apps before trying to get pregnant, in preparation, and found that after a few months of trying, they weren't getting pregnant.

They couldn't understand why, since the app clearly said they were ovulating.

I mean, most women spend most of our adult lives trying to avoid getting pregnant before we're ready, it can't be all that hard right?

Well, as timely as we'd all like to believe our bodies are with this typical 28-day cycle, of course it is no surprise to find out that some of us may not fall into that perfect cycle category.

In that same general thought process, the app will take information you load into it, such as when you get your period, how heavy it might be and the length, amongst other things.

It will do its analysis and estimate when it thinks you are ovulating.

Many women have longer or shorter phases within each cycle, which would either mean you ovulate sooner or later than what the app may estimate.

When paired with other ovulation predicting tools, these apps become an extremely useful and a very important tool.

This chapter is sort of an at-home starter kit in what you can do to further increase your odds of getting pregnant before turning to medications and procedures used in Western medicine.

These are non-invasive, simple ways to help you get pregnant faster.

Ovulation Prediction Kits and Testing Strips

Ovulation prediction kits (OPK) and testing strips are a great way to accurately tell when you are about to ovulate.

These tools are able to detect luteinizing hormone (LH) surges as you near ovulation.

While LH is always present in our bodies, we produce more when we are about to ovulate.

This communicates to our bodies that it's time to release an egg.

The LH surge increases around 24 to 48 hours prior to ovulation.

It may take 2 or 3 cycles for the OPKs to lock down when you are truly ovulating, as not every woman's hormone levels are the same.

The OPKs basically learn the way your body works and predicts ovulation accordingly.

To properly use the kit, you should test only once a day, using the first urination of the day.

Your urine is the most concentrated at that time and the kits and strips can detect the hormones more easily in order to properly tell you if you are nearing ovulation.

Generally speaking, once you get a positive indication of your LH surge beginning, you should plan on having sex for the next 3 days.

Since there are so many different types of OPKs and testing strips, they range from very simple to far more advanced.

I personally prefer ones that are a bit more advanced like the ones made by Clearblue, specifically their Advance Digital option.

This detects not only LH, but also estrogen.

When estrogen levels begin to rise, it displays a flashing smiley face indicating high fertility.

It will continue to display this until it detects your LH surge.

At that point, it will display a static smiley face, indicating peak fertility.

Generally speaking, it's recommended that you have sex every other day when you are in the high fertility phase.

When peak fertility is indicated, you should have sex on that day and the day immediately after.

These are generally able to predict ovulation around 4 or more days prior to the actual egg releasing.

It's possible that the test may not show any LH surge and this likely means that you did not ovulate for that month.

Because they are extremely accurate (about 99%), if you sense that you may have an ovulation issue, it may be a good indicator that you'll want to talk to your doctor sooner than later.

Overall, kits and strips are a cheap and extremely accurate method of predicting ovulation.

I know several friends that got pregnant on their first cycle of using them after months of trying.

Basal Body Temperature Charting

Another accurate ovulation predicting tool is basal body temperature charting (BBT).

BBT is defined as your lowest body temperature within a given 24-hour period.

You can't just use any thermometer to measure, you'll need a basal thermometer.

They are known to be more precise and accurate.

Measuring can either be taken by mouth or by vagina, but either way you should be consistent and not measure using alternating methods.

Just as with OPKs, you should measure your BBT first thing in the morning before your foot even hits the floor to get the most accurate measurement.

Taking your temperature at the same time every morning is also very important for accuracy.

Pre-ovulation, your temperature will likely chart somewhere between 97.2 to 97.7 degrees Fahrenheit.

The day after you ovulate, however, your temperature should raise 0.5 to 1 degree and remain constant until your next period.

If you become pregnant, you will see the temperature maintained at the higher level.

The only negative to this method is that it could take months to accurately predict ovulation but can be a helpful tool if you're willing to be patient.

Cervical Mucus

Another simple way to tell if you're nearing ovulation is through your cervical mucus (CM), also known as vaginal discharge.

I know, I know, we don't usually talk about things like that, but in this case it's actually a really great indicator of ovulation.

The order is usually something like this: you get your period, then you may see none to a light amount of discharge over the next few days, followed by some cloudy and sticky CM, then as you get closer to ovulation the
CM will become thinner, wetter, and stretchier like egg whites.

When you see the egg white mucus start to form, you are in the prime baby making phase.

Our bodies produce this sort of mucus in order to make it easier for the sperm to travel up the cervix to reach the egg.

Just after ovulation, you should observe the mucus decrease and become thicker again.

Sometimes you may be able to see the cervical mucus just by wiping when you go to the bathroom.

If that doesn't work for you, then you may need to check by inserting a clean finger into your vagina to be able to get enough CM to examine.

If there is not enough CM on your finger or very little, then you are more than likely not currently ovulating, as mucus increases during this time.

All of these methods of observation work great alone, but when combining at least 2 or all 3 together, you optimize your chances of timing ovulation correctly.

Timing Intercourse

Once you have an idea of when you should be nearing ovulation, you and your partner should have sex once a day, every other day.

Ideally you should begin this pattern about 5 days before ovulation.

Then on the day you are predicted to ovulate, have sex that day and the day after.

Having sex every other day allows his sperm to regenerate and give you the best soldiers he can possibly give.

Sperm can survive for several days in a woman's body after intercourse, so more sex doesn't necessarily mean better odds.

Having sex more can mean he'll have fewer sperm that could be more immature in his ejaculate and having sex less can mean that the sperm that is being ejaculated may be slower and more abnormal.

An egg only lasts for a maximum of 24 hours in a woman's body if it's not fertilized, so making sure your timing is right is very important.

When using at least 2 of these methods together, you should have no problem timing when to have intercourse properly.

Sex Tips for Conception

While some believe that certain positions help you to get pregnant more easily, data has not proven that yet.

What seems to be a consensus, though, is that gravity can only help the situation.

So as long as you lay flat after sex, that gravitational pull should help at least keep the sperm going in the right direction.

Lie flat immediately after sex for about 15 minutes.

Standing up or going to the bathroom may pull away some sperm that may otherwise have a chance of getting you pregnant.

What can help move the little guys along as well are some personal lubricants.

Most ordinary ones may work against your goal of getting pregnant, so you need to make sure to use ones specifically meant for aiding conception.

I personally like one called Pre-Seed Fertility-Friendly Personal Lubricant.

Before intercourse you use a tube to inject a bit into your vagina near the cervix.

It is meant to mimic your cervical mucus, making it easier for the sperm to travel to the cervix.

Taking Robitussin is also known to thin cervical mucus in order to help move sperm along as well.

Of course, do be aware of drug interactions, but if you are able to take it without issue it may help to get his sperm to your egg.

Another method I recently discovered has helped several couples to get pregnant without medical intervention.

It mimics what a lot of people like to call the turkey baster method.

It's a bit more technical in that it places a cup of your partner's sperm near your cervix to give the little guys the best chance of getting to your egg.

You are to leave the cup in for about 4 to 6 hours after it's inserted.

There are a few different methods of going about doing this, but one in particular has all of the necessary pieces included.

This is called The Stork, OTC.

It is available at several major drug store chains, or you can order it direct online.

The success rate is reported to be the same as procedures like intra uterine inseminations (IUIs) but at a fraction of the cost and without having to visit a doctor.

After intercourse, or using this method, it is also important not to expose yourself to excess heat.

Do not take a bath, go in a hot tub, do strenuous exercises, go in a sauna or anything like it for at least a couple of days during your peak baby making time.

Since sperm can survive for days inside a woman's body, if you expose your body to excess heat, it could damage the sperm.

The same goes for men, during baby making attempts, they should avoid tight underwear, hot baths, laptops, etc.

This part may sound completely obvious, but don't douche after sex.

It will greatly reduce your ability to get pregnant and could put you at risk of a pelvic infection.

More important than anything, try to make it fun.

I know we talked about sex as a form of stress relief earlier and it is, but anyone who has been trying to conceive for even a few months knows that sex can become more of a chore than the fun it should be.

It is so important to your relationship and your mental health to keep it fun and light while still achieving your goals of having a baby.

Try getting out of your comfort zone and shake things up a bit, even if that means morning sex versus only sex at night.

Of course, you can use your imagination on how you can be more adventurous than that!

Chances are you'll have less sex when kids are around, so take advantage of your free time now!

Chapter 8: The Western System

Western Medicine: Where to Begin

"There's no telling how many miles you have to run while chasing a dream." – Anonymous

Sometimes it takes a village to have AND raise a family.

There is nothing wrong with asking for help.

By now you may have been trying to conceive for months, maybe even years and you're thinking about going to see a specialist.

The thought of undergoing Western fertility treatments can be overwhelming.

With so few people talking about their experiences, you may feel like you're the only one approaching your doctor to discuss a potential fertility issue.

The fear of not knowing what to expect, what sort of treatments you'll have to undergo, how long it may take to get pregnant, it's all so intimidating to think of.

Just know, you are NOT alone and seeking out professional help is nothing to be afraid or ashamed of.

There are a lot of us out there.

It's important to know where and when to begin.

This next chapter will dive into the preliminary phases of selecting a fertility specialist and what to consider.

When to Call the Doctor

Believe it or not, but trying to conceive can take up to a year for an average couple to get pregnant.

As a general guideline, if you are under 35 years of age and you've been trying to get pregnant for over a year, it may be time to consult with a doctor.

For women over 35, the general guideline for when it's time to see a fertility doctor is when you've been trying for 6 months.

After 40 years of age, it is recommended that you see a reproductive endocrinologist immediately.

I personally recommend seeing your physician and/or OBGYN before even trying, when you know you are ready.

It's good to get a full check-up including a blood draw and general physical when you are thinking about getting pregnant.

Simple issues that any physician should be able to diagnose such as thyroid diseases can be huge inhibitors to you getting pregnant.

Diagnosing and treating conditions like that can mean the difference of getting pregnant right away and taking months, even years.

If you already know you have certain medical conditions that could affect your ability to get pregnant, you should talk to a doctor immediately.

Multiple miscarriages, thyroid disease, endometriosis, diabetes, polycystic ovarian syndrome, certain STDs and many more diagnoses can have a negative effect on your fertility if not treated properly.

Certain medications can also affect your fertility, some may surprise you.

If you are taking certain sinus medication, psychiatric medication, NSAIDs (non-steroidal anti-inflammatory drugs), blood pressure medications, diuretics, steroids, epilepsy mediations, thyroid medications, chemotherapy or skin lotions and serums with hormones, then you need to discuss your intention or attempts at getting pregnant with your doctor.

I want to note that it would be impossible to list all medications here that could affect fertility, but you should talk to your doctor about anything and everything you are taking (over-the-counter and prescription).

Nothing is too small.

They may need to prescribe you an alternative medication that won't interfere with your efforts to get pregnant.

Even in the absence of medications or a diagnosed condition interfering, certain symptoms indicate possible fertility issues, so pay attention to your body and talk to your doctor if you've experienced or are currently experiencing any of the following:

- Heavy and/or prolonged menstruation
- Irregular or absent menstruation
- Painful menstruation
- Severe acne
- Excessive body and/or facial hair
- Hair loss
- Chronic pelvic pain

Listen to your body, I mean really listen.

Symptoms that you wouldn't normally expect to be attached to a condition that might affect fertility could be the answer to a quicker diagnosis.

It's EXTREMELY important to mention everything, even if you think it's trivial and unrelated.

A couple that my husband and I are friends with spent over 5 years trying to get pregnant.

She would have pelvic pain around the time she thought she was ovulating and had painful menstruation.

She brushed off the symptoms and didn't think twice about mentioning to her doctor because she figured it was all pretty normal.

After 3 IUIs, her doctor sat her down to discuss IVF as the next option.

During her exam, they noticed some fluid buildup on her ultrasound.

Her doctor found this curious and scheduled laparoscopic surgery to see if she possibly had endometriosis.

This was something she NEVER considered.

Once she began to read up on the condition, she was surprised to see how many of the symptoms lined up with what she had felt.

Well, low and behold, it turned out she had a severe case of endometriosis.

Her doctor cleared away a lot of the scarring and additional tissue during the laparoscopic surgery and within a month they were ready to get to trying again.

They scheduled one more IUI and they were finally able to get pregnant!

After all those years, they were blessed with twins, a boy and a girl.

If she and her doctor had a better dialogue about her symptoms, maybe they would have caught this earlier and she would have avoided years of frustration.

This sort of thing should be diagnosed before you even have to see a fertility specialist, but is often times missed.

If you've experienced any of the above-mentioned symptoms or you've been diagnosed with any of these conditions, it's extremely important to talk to your doctor in advance of trying to get pregnant so that you can prepare your body to carry a baby.

Have an open dialogue and again, be thorough in your explanation of your symptoms.

You can potentially save yourself additional time, stress, and heartache.

This was my story too, in fact this couple helped change our path.

Their story got me thinking and doing my own research.

I'd previously mentioned my symptoms that are perfectly in line with endometriosis to my first OBGYN, especially one in particular (painful bowel movements during menstruation – I know, sorry TMI, but it's important to mention).

She brushed it off and basically made me feel as though I was crazy.

I thought, well she's the expert, I guess what I'm feeling is just part of my menstrual cycle, so I brushed it off and put it to the back of my mind.

This experience was when I was in my early 20s.

Over 10 years later, my friend's diagnosis got me thinking about my symptoms again.

I did some research online and it did seem to point toward endometriosis.

Was this all in my head, though?

Am I just a hypochondriac that's learned about this issue with my friend and I'm just trying to find something wrong with myself?

My husband, Mr. Cynic, was surprisingly steadfast in his belief that I should mention having the same surgery to my doctor since my symptoms seemed to point directly to endometriosis.

We were met with hesitation at first from our doctor, as she did agree that the symptoms were in line with endometriosis, however she felt that they weren't severe enough to warrant surgery.

She thought that even if I did have endometriosis that it wouldn't interfere with my ability to get pregnant.

Well, after a failed attempt at IVF number 1, we decided this was too important to ignore.

A few months had passed and I continued to mention the surgery to my doctor.

She eventually relented and agreed to do the surgery.

As it would turn out, the surgery helped us to discover that I had advanced stage 3 endometriosis (out of 4 stages).

As happy as I was to finally get a real diagnosis, I was also extremely saddened and a bit angry that this wasn't something that was found 10 years earlier.

Ultimately, looking on the bright side, I could now finally get the treatment I really needed.

I just wish that I'd adopted my current philosophy and pressed for this sooner.

By the way, 50% of women being treated for infertility have endometriosis.

It's crazy to think that something so prevalent in the infertility community is overlooked so often, for so long.

I'll say it again, it is extremely important to push for what you know is right for you to get a clear diagnosis sooner than later.

And while the assumption is that fertility issues usually typically lie with women, an easy initial step is having your partner also do a quick check-up with his doctor.

I would also suggest having your partner do a semen analysis early on.

It's an easy, quick, and relatively cheap test (through insurance of course).

If there is an issue with his sperm, then that should help narrow down a treatment plan significantly and possibly avoid unnecessary and invasive testing and treatments for you.

I know for my husband and I, I initiated testing earlier than was suggested by our doctors, but still hadn't thought about it prior to subjecting myself to some fertility treatments.

We went through 4 rounds of clomiphene citrate (pre-diagnosis) before I even requested the semen analysis with our doctor.

It turns out that his tests came back completely normal, but had the results come back different, the ovulation medication would likely have done us no good.

Long story short, do some basic testing for the both of you before you begin any fertility medications or any invasive testing...

and make sure you are very forthcoming with your symptoms.

Nothing is too small or insignificant, even if someone along the way may have convinced you otherwise.

Choosing the Right Doctor

Once you've decided that it's time to see a fertility specialist, it's important to make sure you are choosing the right one.

Don't hurry into any decisions because you feel rushed for time.

I know it can feel like a bomb is about to go off and you need to get pregnant before that happens.

But just think about it, if you choose the wrong doctor, you could waste far more time.

Each month is 1 chance to get pregnant for a regular cycle, with certain fertility treatments it's much longer.

For IVF, if you're doing a frozen embryo transfer, between egg retrieval and the embryo transfer process combined, just 1 cycle will take 5 months sometimes (my first looked like this – 1 month for retrieval, skip 1 month for recovery, 2 months of birth control, 1 month of medications to prepare your body for the transfer).

Long story short, choosing the right doctor can mean a lot of time lost.

Personally, I started with good ol' Mr. Google.

Using websites like www.healthgrades.com or www.ratemds.com are very helpful.

They are widely used and their review system is very thorough.

My fertility center and two of their doctors were at the top of the list for my area, so that helped me narrow down my selections.

Another great way to vet your clinic is to review their success rates versus the national average.

The Center for Disease Control (CDC) shares this information.

Although their website isn't exactly up to date, it should give you a good idea of what to expect from the clinics you are looking at.

Another helpful website is www.sart.org.

The Society for Assisted Reproductive Technology (SART) provides statistical data for their list of SART member clinics.

These are great resources to help with your search.

Unfortunately, like myself and for most women, because fertility issues are such a stigma, we don't often share information about our experiences very easily.

I was so afraid to ask anyone for recommendations, I felt so ashamed that we were in this position.

I was so sure that I was the only one in the world that I knew dealing with this and even if I wasn't, I didn't want to "bother" anyone else that I knew was dealing with infertility as well.

If I didn't want to talk about it, they probably wouldn't either.

It was only after I had been going to my reproductive endocrinologist for a few months that I found a friend that was going to the same center and it was only after our husbands ran into each other dropping off *ahemmm* samples.

Further into my treatment, I found out about 2 other friends that were also being treated at the same place, at the same time.

Looking back at my experiences and how good I felt "coming clean" about going through infertility, it really blows my mind to think about how many women are afraid to talk about their experiences.

If talking about it openly means that it could help even one person to know the right places to go and what to look for in a clinic or doctor, then it's all worth it to me.

If you're not quite there yet, then another great resource and starting place in finding the right reproductive doctor for you is through your OBGYN or physician.

You will have already discussed potential fertility issues with them and more often than not, they are the first line of defense and work closely with one another.

I'd already been going to my fertility doctor for a few months by the time my husband was being treated for his cancer, but his oncologist actually recommended my doctor to me.

Since men and women of younger ages that have been diagnosed with cancer and recommended to freeze eggs or sperm before undergoing cancer treatments, they too work closely with reproductive centers.

This was reaffirmation that I'd made the right choice in my clinic.

Asking doctors that you trust and, if you are comfortable enough, asking friends you may know have had some experience with infertility are always some of the best ways to find the right doctor for you.

As happy as I was to find that I made the right choice through Google, my uncertainty if I'd made the right choice were affirmed time and time again through continued conversation.

Once you've narrowed down your options, do a little more recon on the doctors and clinics.

Again, this could mean the difference in getting pregnant next month or in a few years, so choose wisely.

It may seem obvious, but most of us are so overwhelmed with the thought of moving on to fertility treatments that it might be easy to forget these important, basic things that should first be confirmed:

- Are they board certified?
- How long have they been practicing?
- What are their areas of specialization?
- Are they part of a well-respected clinic?

Often, these sorts of things are published online, so you should be able to find out fairly easily.

If you can't find the information online, then don't be afraid to ask for proof while you are at your first visit or call the office.

Does the clinic have a good response time?

It may seem trivial at first, but think about it.

You are going to go through testing and treatments that you will be waiting on follow-up for.

Not only that, but trust me, you will have A LOT of questions.

You want to make sure they are quick to respond, are patient with you and take enough time with you to thoroughly address your concerns.

Now bedside manner, in my opinion, isn't that important.

So, if you are reading reviews and peoples' comments are about their poor attitude, but they have high success rates, then frankly, who the heck cares?

Yes, we may need some petting through this emotional process, but I don't think that's a necessary part of your doctor's job.

Personally, I'd rather get the job done than worry about that.

If that, however, is an important quality for you in your care, then don't settle.

This is your experience and you can always find a doctor that has it all, so make sure you are getting the best care that suits you.

Do they offer the most state of the art technology?

You want to make sure everything they are practicing is the absolute best and newest technology offered.

You of course will go in hoping and maybe expecting to get pregnant right away, and that is of course the hope, but like with anything, expect the best, but prepare for the worst.

Do your homework.

If you don't already have a diagnosis, then research all treatment options that the clinic has to offer.

Assume that you will likely have to undergo IVF, which is usually the end of the line as far as fertility treatments go.

Something that served as a great source of frustration for my husband and I was that new technology for genetic testing was being used elsewhere, but had not yet adopted by our clinic.

Our first round of IVF resulted in 1 normal embryo and 4 abnormal embryos, which was a pretty big shock, considering that we thought we were otherwise normal, pretty healthy early 30 somethings.

After that round's transfer of the normal embryo didn't implant, we met with our doctor to discuss our next options.

It was then, only a few months later that our doctor told us about new genetic testing technology that they were using.

This testing would allow them to see mosaicisms in embryos that previously would have otherwise been placed in the abnormal category.

Mosaic embryos, depending on what abnormalities exist, may result in a healthy pregnancy and completely healthy baby.

My stomach dropped.

Why would something that existed as a method of testing not have been available to us?

We had 5 embryos the last time, surely at least 1 more might have been mosaic.

That was maybe 1 more chance for us to have a healthy baby, possibly even the 2 we'd always dreamt of having.

Not only that, but let's not forget the $10,000 or more in each additional round, stress on my mind, my body, my relationship.

What procedures do their doctors do in house?

Speaking of high costs, you are likely to spend a lot more money out of pocket if you go to a clinic that doesn't do in house procedures.

That was another big reason why I chose my clinic.

They do all of their major procedures in house and have a new, state of the are surgery center at their main location.

If any of the clinics you are considering do their procedures in a hospital, it's likely that each procedure can cost considerably more (roughly 45-60%) than somewhere that does it in their own facility.

The reason for this is that a hospital's overhead is much higher.

This is because of things like having 24-hour staffing and emergency rooms that cannot turn patients without insurance away.

Hospitals end up absorbing these costs when the patients cannot, and in turn, make the costs on patients like you and I much higher.

Obviously, if the procedure is more involved, your doctor's office may choose to do some away in a hospital, so don't be discouraged if they tell you they do some procedures in house and some away.

This is because they are better equipped in case any emergent issues arise.

Just make sure to ask which procedures are done in house or in a hospital and why.

Do they truly listen to and consider your concerns?

You know your body better than anyone else.

One of my most important pieces of advice is to vet this part of your doctor's practice if at all possible.

Even if it means going in for a couple of initial visits to feel them out, at least you wouldn't have wasted years on trusting that they are the experts and to ignore your own voiced concerns.

As I mentioned earlier, I voiced concerns to multiple doctors over the course of more than 10 years and I was all but ignored on multiple occasions.

As thorough as my doctor was, nothing about what I was telling her of my fears of having endometriosis made her feel it was worth putting me through a surgery to explore.

It wasn't until I really pushed and insisted on laparoscopic surgery that I finally got my diagnosis.

Maybe another doctor would have found this sooner, maybe not, who knows, but I feel that it certainly shouldn't have taken multiple doctors over the course of a decade to figure it out.

I can't change the past now, but I can help you to change your path.

In the end, you have to trust that you are getting the best care possible.

If you don't feel that way, you shouldn't be afraid to change fertility clinics or doctors in the same practice.

This is your journey, so don't live in fear of disappointing someone else.

I'll say it again…BE YOUR OWN CHAMPION.

If there is one message you take away from this (and I certainly hope you get much more), please take that away.

Don't feel like you are just a number in their book and they aren't really concerned over your care.

The number one message I've gotten from those that have undergone years of fertility treatments have all said the same.

They wished they'd pushed harder for better care, whatever that meant to their particular case.

One wished she'd asked for more frequent scans to diagnose a condition that was found years into her treatment.

One wished she got more one on one time with her doctor.

I wished I'd pushed harder for a diagnosis sooner, but it all comes down to one thing.

Making sure you are taking care of number one, YOU, and that your care team is doing the same.

Chapter 9: The Scissor Program

More Cost Saving Secrets: What Your Doctor Probably Isn't Telling You

"What feels like the end is often the beginning." – Anonymous

More often than not, those undergoing fertility treatments are probably expecting their doctors' offices to present them with options that will lessen their financial burdens.

I can speak directly to this, but my fertility clinic did not mention anything of the sort to me.

Maybe it's because my insurance policy partially covered costs or they just figured we could afford it financially, who knows.

Ultimately, they are there for one reason, to help make a baby…

…and let's be honest, it is a business and they need to make money, so your financial burden isn't really their first priority.

Not to say that I blame them, I don't, I do however think we all have a responsibility to seek out information to protect ourselves.

There are so many options available to us that aren't openly advertised.

So, I figure, I'll help to make it a little easier on you and let you know about everything I know now about how to save a little or a lot of money on what can be an extremely expensive process.

Grants and Scholarships

Sound weird that there are scholarships and grants that assist in fertility treatments, right?

That is reserved for schooling usually.

Well in this case, they work pretty similarly to the way grants and scholarships work for funding education.

Both require certain minimal criteria and you must apply to receive them.

Minimally they require some personal information, like your name, address, and dates of birth (for you and your partner).

They also require financial information, so that they can make sure that they aren't funding a greedy millionaire's treatments, but instead to people who truly are in need.

So, they expect proof of your previous income levels through tax documents over the last few years.

Once approved for a grant, the foundation will provide a certain level of approved cash to go toward your treatment or treatments.

Scholarships work a bit differently.

The foundation that supplies the scholarship will likely work with certain fertility centers and have treatments at that center donated to you.

Some require application fees, so if you feel relatively sure that you should be eligible based off of their criteria, then it may be well worth it.

Some grants or scholarships I've seen will pay for treatments upwards of $16,000.

Most, though, hover around the $10,000 range.

I won't list the available programs here, as they may change over the years, but if you do a search for fertility scholarships or fertility grants, you will have no problem finding them.

IVF Refund Program

Now these programs really piqued my interest when I first learned about them.

I was surprised that my fertility clinic hadn't offered this as an option to my husband and I after our first round of IVF, once we'd exhausted our insurance coverage.

The IVF Refund Program (which can go by other names including the Shared Risk Program, depending on where it's offered) offers to partially or fully refund your money if IVF isn't successful to those who are paying fully out of pocket.

They usually do not offer the program to those 40 and over around and will typically only approve patients that they anticipate will have success.

Most programs offer this to qualifying patients who pay for up to 6 rounds of IVF (or even more in some places) upfront.

When payment is made in advance the program may offer some discounted pricing.

There is, however, a catch.

Even if you are enrolled in a program that offers a full refund, you may still be hit with some "fees" that will offset what you get back.

Various costs included in these fees may include things like anesthesia, pre-screening (blood and ultrasound), office visits, or fertility medications.

Conversely, if you are successful, paying upfront may end up meaning you pay more than what you may have otherwise if paid for individually.

Overall, many couples choose to partake in these programs for more peace of mind.

Even if they end up paying more per round in the end, at least they know that if they don't find success in the process that they aren't left for broke.

Also, read the fine print.

What is their definition of a successful cycle?

Is it a positive pregnancy test or a live birth?

If you get a positive pregnancy test, but miscarry soon after, the program may consider that a "successful cycle."

Is the treatment plan more aggressive than usual?

This could be a negative, in that you may be put at a higher risk level so that the clinic can try to get you pregnant faster.

The program will either be offered directly through your clinic or possibly through a 3rd party vendor (if at all).

Before you decide to sign up, get as much information from them as possible so that you can make an educated decision as to whether it would be a good fit for you.

If you feel that you will have a good chance of success with your first round of IVF, then the program may not be right for you.

Pharmaceutical Assistance Programs

Somewhere around half of us getting fertility treatments don't have any financial assistance from insurance for our specialty medications.

These are where a large amount of the costs for fertility treatments come from.

Pharmaceutical assistance programs offer financial assistance in the form of discounted medications.

Again, like with grants and scholarships, there is an application where you have to provide the same sort of information including tax returns to show that there is a financial need for their assistance.

You must be fully self-paying for the medications in order to be eligible.

If you are about to undergo chemotherapy and you are freezing your eggs prior to treatment, a wide range of financial assistance is offered to you, but you have to be sure to apply prior to any fertility treatments.

The window is often tight between diagnosis and treatment, so you have to be sure to act quickly.

Currently, in the U.S., the Compassionate Care and DesignRX programs seem to be the most prominent.

They offer a range of assistance, depending on where they feel your needs are, anywhere from 5% to 75% in medicinal discounts.

Coupons

Another simple way to save some money on your specialty medications is through coupons.

It's such a simple thing, but so many of us don't even know there are coupons for these medications or simply forget to even look.

Websites like www.goodrx.com offer some discounts, although likely smaller than what some of these other programs may offer.

The positive, though, is that they are offered to everyone, no income check, no signing up.

Doreen, 39, used a coupon for one of her specialty medications that would have otherwise cost her $250, but instead she got it for free.

Some may only save you a few dollars, but hey, with the amount of medications you may have to use, that could add up to a nice dinner really quickly and you might really need a few of those!

Overseas Medications

When insurance coverage is either exhausted or it was never an option at all, and you find that you aren't eligible to receive grants or scholarships, you'll need to buy your specialty medications out of pocket.

For me, insurance covered about ¾ or so of my medications from the first round of IVF, and that's for a lifetime maximum, not "oh it'll start over next year," that's all you get.

That was a huge shock to me, I cried for a while when I realized that I'd hit the limit with my insurance.

Your doctor's office will likely point you in the direction of one or two specialty pharmacies that they trust and often work with, but know that there are more options.

One of which, I wished I'd looked into earlier is getting your medications online from an overseas location.

Medications can be a third of the cost that they are in U.S. specialty pharmacies.

More trusted sources are medications shipped from either Israel or England.

The reason the medications cost significantly less here are because these countries' governments have price limits on what those medications can be sold for.

My husband, the risk taker and money saver of the family, was the first to bring this up and I was fully against it initially.

I wanted to vet the online pharmacies and their facilities.

More importantly, I wanted to know what my doctor's opinion of the whole thing was.

Well, she was all for it, to my surprise, with the caveat that they come from somewhere that required a prescription and was located in a country that has strict drug regulations (like the two listed above).

If you do decide to go this route, you should also be sure that you know alternative names for medications (like generic ones).

Often times, the names are a bit different, but generally are listed under their generic names.

They also come in specific quantities, so if you need only 4 vials of something, you may have to buy it in a pack of 5 since that might be all they offer.

Overall, even with some extra, you'll still end up spending significantly less.

You will also need to order with a few weeks of lead time, so if you know you will begin IVF treatments a month from now, you will need to start the process today.

They generally ask for 4 weeks' time in order to get the medication shipped over to you.

Remember, everyone's body reacts differently to the fertility medications, so what your doctor's office asks you to order upfront may not be completely accurate with what you'll need in the end.

You may order too much, or not enough.

They will test your levels throughout the process and if the medication isn't doing what it's supposed to, you may need to order more.

If you need to order more on a moment's notice, then you won't be able to order the additional needed medications from your overseas pharmacy.

Specialty pharmacies in your area will either have the medications on hand for immediate fill or they can be shipped to your home within 24 hours (permitting it's not over a weekend).

It will obviously cost you more to get it locally, but at least you were able to save on what you could.

Shop Specialty Pharmacies

If you are still uncomfortable with the idea of using an overseas pharmacy, then it's important to note that specialty pharmacies may have varying costs.

As I mentioned before, if you are paying out of pocket, your doctor's office will more than likely point you in the direction of one or two specialty pharmacies that they typically work with.

It's important to know that you have multiple options (at home, not overseas) available to you.

So before just taking your doctor's recommendations, make sure that you're shopping around.

Prices are relatively similar typically, but just like with coupons, even slight differences in the amount of medications you need for each treatment can add up quickly.

Also, make sure to mention that you are paying out of pocket, they may offer further discounts for that.

An additional discount that is often offered is for patients of specific fertility clinics, so make sure to mention that in your order as well.

Specialty pharmacies will often work with you and may have additional money saving programs available if you just ask.

Medical Tourism

If getting your medications from overseas didn't freak you out, then this section might also speak to you.

The idea of being treated for things like IVF overseas might not be right for everyone, but there are other countries that may be more advanced than where you are located at a far lesser cost.

I know, novel idea, right? Your country isn't the best at everything??

It is important, as usual, to make sure you do extremely thorough research and make sure you are choosing locations wisely.

An international organization called Joint Commission International (JCI) "works to improve patient safety and quality of health care in the international community by offering education, publications, advisory services, and international accreditation and certification."

This agency works to give accreditations to various hospitals and medical centers around the world, enabling patients to feel safer in choosing facilities that abide by higher standards.

There are also many medical tourism agencies that may be located in your area that offer assistance in finding the right care team for your needs.

Pre-Genetic Testing

Pre-Genetic Testing (PGT – also known as Pre-Genetic Screening or PGS), is commonly used in patients to choose to test their embryos prior to freezing for possible chromosomal issues.

The testing is also able to identify gender, but that's just a fun extra.

For my husband and I, we wanted to do PGT, mostly because we wanted to make sure that we were transferring healthy embryos but partially because we wanted to know the genders too.

Well, it's a good thing we did it because, even though it does cost a pretty penny (often times averaging around $1,000-$2,000), we saved ourselves time, grief, physical stress, and money in the end.

The reason that I say this is because (as I mentioned earlier) of 5 embryos, 4 came back as chromosomally abnormal.

After reading about the specific abnormalities our embryos had, the likelihood that I would have had a full-term pregnancy with any of the 4 were nil.

So that means, I would have subjected myself to 4 times the fertility hormones to prepare my body for each transfer, 4 times the physical and emotional stress, not knowing why they didn't work.

Each transfer would have taken approximately a month, not to mention the dreaded 2-week wait after that.

If pregnancy wasn't achieved, the clinic typically asks for you to wait for another cycle to pass before you begin pumping yourself with medications again.

That means for 1 transfer, you're waiting a minimum of 2 months, maybe 3.

Imagine that times 4, and what would have ended in 5 in my case, since my 1 "normal" embryo didn't take.

That also would have meant 5 times as much cost in fertility medications, ultrasounds, blood work, check-ups, embryo storage and transfer costs.

In the end, that would have added up to much more than the $1,000-$2,000 we spent in PGT.

I honestly believe that nobody would regret deciding to do this testing.

Max Out That FSA

If you have a Flexible Spending Account (FSA) through your insurance, make sure that you are using it to its maximum benefit.

My FSA maxed out at $6,000 for the year and I knew that round 2 of IVF was coming, so I made sure to request the full $6,000.

I had easily used that full $6,000 within the first half of the year, who am I kidding, it was the first quarter.

For those unfamiliar with FSAs, they are funded with pre-tax income.

Basically, it means that you will save what you would have paid in taxes on the money set aside to pay those medical expenses.

Depending on your income level, that could mean a discount anywhere from 10% to 37%.

Tax Deductions

If the fertility treatments you are undergoing exceed 10% of your adjusted gross income, then you're in luck!

In the U.S., the IRS will allow medical expenses to be deducted.

That means you can deduct things like your check-up costs, lab fees, medications, ultrasounds, and bloodwork.

If you live a decent distance away from your clinic, they may even allow deductions on your travel expenses including hotel stays and meals!

I would have never even imagined submitting those sorts of expenses to my accountant, but it's important that you keep receipts from every bit of your expenses in the process.

Your accountant can help unlock hidden savings and get you some money back!

Check Your Insurance Lifetime Maximum

Something that I discovered the hard way was that my insurance had a small lifetime maximum.

I didn't think twice about checking alternative insurance plans that may have had better benefits until it was too late and I was stuck with the decision I'd made the year prior.

My lifetime maximum for pharmaceutical benefits was $10,000, and while I was 100% appreciative that I got anything...

...since I know many couples don't get anything AT ALL...

...I was still a bit saddened that I wasn't more informed or aware of the fact that I had better options available to me that could have saved us tens of thousands of dollars more.

Your work likely offers multiple plans, so make sure you are checking the details of them.

Some offer much higher lifetime maximums, which will save you greatly in the end if you end up having to do multiple rounds of IVF.

Programs like Optum (offered through United Healthcare) help you navigate through the complex nature of the fertility game.

They help to find you the best resources for care and assist in reducing your costs where possible, whether through their prescription (RX) program or through their Care program.

There are several programs just like this, this is just one example of the possibilities that are offered to you.

The first step to saving money is to arm yourself with the knowledge of what options that are offered to you.

Accepting

Chapter 11: Interview with an Acupuncturist/Chinese Medicine Practitioner

"Change your thoughts and you change your world." – Norman Vincent Pearle

Stephanie Bartolotti is my acupuncturist, she owns and runs a wonderful clinic near me called New Direction Natural Medicine.

When you enter her office, you're met with soothing fragrances coming from their essential oil diffuser, light, calming music, an organic tea and water station, comfortable seating and a sweet receptionist that tends to your needs right away.

This creates the perfect start to the relaxing experience to come.

After one of my treatments, Stephanie was kind enough to sit down with me for a bit and share her experiences and knowledge in Chinese Medicine as it relates to infertility.

Here is what she had to share:

Stephanie: So, I've been practicing nine years.

Most of what I treat would be infertility, anxiety, women's health, and pain. Patients tend to gravitate toward me for these main few things.

I think ultimately why I wanted to get into healthcare was because growing up I had a lot of health issues.

I had issues with my eyes where I had to wear glasses, I got surgery and even had to wear and eye patch at times. was diagnosed with scoliosis.

I had a back brace for 10 years and had to do a lot of deep tissue massages, which were pretty brutal on me.

I just thought, there's got to be a better way than torturing people, you know?

So, what ultimately got me into acupuncture, specifically, was that I started as a massage therapist and I did that for six years.

I wanted to help patients in a bigger capacity, so I decided to go the massage therapy route.

On my first day of massage, somebody said, "Get out now. You don't want to be doing this the rest of your life."

And I said, "Okay" (with a laugh).

That really stuck in my head, you know?

And I knew just with my body, that it wasn't going to be good long term, it's a shorter career span anyways for massage.

So, I decided to try and take a course in acupuncture, and the teacher was AMAZING.

I took the course at Everglades University, where they do a Bachelor's Degree in Alternative Medicine (it should be noted that

Everglades University has various traditional collegiate programs and does not lean toward non-traditional, alternative degrees).

I was always interested in that field because I grew up doing ballet to get out of my back brace, and I always wanted to take care of my body and be healthy.

I wanted to do anything I could do to be healthy and be able to maintain the ballet career.

So, anyway, I took the course, and they did a demo on the dean of the school.

She had horrible sciatica, which made her walk with a cane.

She did acupuncture and just like that, her pain was gone.

She was walking around after her treatment without her cane, so I was pretty blown away.

A lot of the people in my class actually left there and went to acupuncture school because the teacher was so influential.

They didn't really like her too much at that school because of it!

Kim: Wow, that's crazy how you got here.

Thanks for going over that.

I always like to know the how and why you chose such a unique career path.

Now on to the more formal questions!

As far as treatments in Chinese Medicine go, can you explain how it pairs well with Western treatments and how they complement one another?

Stephanie: Yeah, so, several studies have been done that show some really impressive statistics.

One in particular studied patients going through IVF treatments.

The study compared women in 2 control groups.

One group of women were going through IVF with the traditional medications and the other control group included women going through IVF, but these women added in acupuncture pre and post embryo transfer.

With IVF only, 26.3% resulted in pregnancy, while the group doing acupuncture just pre and post embryo transfer rose to 42.5% that resulted in pregnancy.

That's a significant difference, nearly doubled.

The statistics are similar while using Chinese herbs for fertility versus drug therapy, again results are approximately twice as successful.

So just that speaks for itself, and this doesn't even include leading up to that time because some people will read research and say, "Oh,

I'll just do it before and after because that's going to increase my chances."

But this study is showing the statistics of just doing it before and after the embryo transfer.

If you're doing it way before you're going to do your treatments, anywhere between 3 to 6 months prior to treatment, your results are going to be much better than that.

I recommend to patients anywhere from 3 to 6 months to get their body prepared to try to conceive, because you want your body to be in the most optimal state.

You want your period to be regular, you want all these processes to happen in order to make you more fertile.

So of course, women don't want to wait.

They don't want to hear, "Oh, I have to wait an extra length of time."

Because they've already been waiting and they're already frustrated and they want it yesterday, you know?

Kim: Hi, that's me (I say with a laugh)!

Stephanie: So yeah, that's the hard part because a lot of times people come in just like, "I just want the IVF and I want to have it now."

But being more patient and getting your body where it needs to be obviously is going to give you the ideal situation so that you can conceive.

Kim: So, then for women undergoing fertility treatments or are generally looking to get pregnant, what treatments do you most commonly use?

Stephanie: So, of course it depends on if you're doing IVF, or just trying naturally, or doing IUI.

For everyone, it's going to be acupuncture and herbs.

If someone is doing all the IVF drugs, even though the studies show the herbs are complementary and they do increase chances, a lot of doctors are afraid of herbs, and they don't recommend using them during treatments.

But I did have a patient that was open to doing Chinese herbs with IVF, so she didn't tell her doctors, and she got pregnant.

She'd done two cycles prior to that that weren't successful.

But a lot of the doctors, like I said, don't want patients to take herbs just because they don't have the knowledge or the training in it and they're scared because they've heard things that aren't true.

For most people, though, my protocol is acupuncture and herbs.

For most women, it's a poor blood flow issue and stress is also a big factor.

I also see a lot of women with painful periods or clotty periods, cysts, endometriosis, fibroids and PCOS.

So, if there's poor blood flow in the reproductive organs, then that's what forms the cysts and the fibroids and all those things that get in the way of implanting.

So that's the first thing I try to do, is to kind of clean everything out and make the environment ideal for the baby to attach and conceive and to have a healthy pregnancy.

Kim: What else would you use treatments like this for?

Stephanie: Acupuncture does a lot of things.

It stimulates the HPOA access, which is Hypothalamic Pituitary Ovarian Adrenal access.

I know that's a whole big term, but it basically helps to regulate hormones such as LH and FSH.

It's going to improve circulation in the reproductive system so that those organs are functioning better overall, it's going to help to reduce stress, which is linked to infertility and can definitely be a factor.

It can improve egg quality, for men, it can improve sperm, both in motility and morphology, which are things that Western doctors don't really have an answer for.

To treat that, I use herbs because herbs are going to be really complementary.

It's addressing the internal issues, and then acupuncture pairs really well with it.

You're always going to get better results combining the 2, but it's just dependent on the individual patient and what they have going on.

So, basically if somebody doesn't really have any explanation as to why they couldn't conceive or they haven't tried for too long, it wouldn't be as aggressive with their treatments as compared to someone that has a lot of fibroids and horrible endometriosis, or they've been trying for a really long time, things like that.

And then if somebody is on a schedule, of, "This is when I'm doing IVF, this is when I'm doing IUI," I'm going to work with that too.

So, it's kind of just dependent on where the patient is at, I kind of meet them where they're at, but also be realistic about, "This is what it's going to take. This is the ideal scenario."

Kim: So, for those who are going through fertility treatments or just wanting to get pregnant, what's the most important thing you could do outside of coming here at home to help to up your chances of conceiving?

Stephanie: Anything they can do to manage stress is really important.

Whatever that is for somebody, whatever is meditative for them.

Not necessarily sitting there and doing the whole "Om" thing, you know, but some people find painting or drawing meditative.

Maybe knitting or sewing, things like that.

Anything you find that reduces stress that is meditative to you.

Diet is really also important, eating good food.

That's why I always give handouts to patients with foods they should eat.

So, eggs are one of the really good foods.

You obviously want organic, free range, pastured eggs.

There are a lot of different foods that I recommend for fertility, and there's a few books written on those foods as well.

Eating good quality, grass fed meats are good, beets, eggplants, things that are going to help with blood.

There's eating organic, healthy, staying away from the sugar and processed foods.

And traditionally, if you get any old chicken versus the free range, organic, then you're going to get hormones and antibiotics and things that can screw up your hormones.

And then another thing would be to stay away from plastics and microwave things, because they emit estrogens and chemicals.

Kim: I completely agree.

I try to live my life in that way, I've practiced this for years prior to my attempts at getting pregnant, so at least I had that going for me!

I used to get crazy acid reflux, was prescribed a million different medications that basically did nothing and decided let me just try eating organic, clean foods.

Pretty soon after, my acid reflux was significantly reduced, so much so that I only now get it when I indulge in certain foods.

So, next I have a question from my husband.

He was wondering, for those who can't necessarily afford the treatments, is there anything you would say from a Chinese medicine perspective that they can do themselves at home, aside from just what you were mentioning?

Stephanie: It's hard to say because I always do an evaluation on the patient to see, and obviously my tool is Chinese medicine.

I'd say the biggest thing would be, again, the diet and the stress.

Those are the main two big factors.

And as far as the prices, I mean, it's way cheaper than the IVF treatments, as you know.

And it is an investment, and that's kind of one of the frustrating things in medicine because people aren't used to paying for their healthcare because they have insurance, but they are paying for it.

Insurance is very expensive, so for some people, it's hard to think of paying outside of that, but the results are there.

Because health insurance is good for emergencies, for sure, but as far as chronic issues and things, they're going to give you a drug to mask the symptoms, they're not really going to help you get better.

It's sick care, it's not really healthcare.

So, it is like the best investment that you can make, and once patients go through the course of treatment, I have the baby pictures, and I get the testimonials and all these things, it's totally worth it, and it's actually cheap in the long run.

Kim: So, for those who are just starting their journey and have now decided that they're wanting to move on to Chinese medicine, is there anything you wish your patients knew going into the process that would make your job easier, or the treatments more effective.

Stephanie: I'd say lifestyle is the biggest thing.

Years ago, I had some patients that were in their late 40s, and they had super high stress, super crappy diet, and worked way too many hours.

I mean, in that case, I would have to have a magic wand.

So that's the biggest thing is they have to be committed and take it seriously because if they don't, they're fighting against the results that they could get.

So being in a place where they're ready to sacrifice.

I took a seminar a while ago on advanced maternal age, so older women trying to conceive, and if they couldn't have a baby, how to deal with that.

And it was interesting, they were talking about what it is that you're looking for to fulfill with that child?

And if someone couldn't conceive due to their age and other things, how could that be fulfilled in another way?

It was very interesting and introspective, "Okay, why do I really want this and how would I feel having this? And is there something else in my life that could fulfill that?"

I have a patient, she's working 14-hour days, she was eating once a day, she was really overweight, eating crappy food, and sodas, and things like that.

I'm not a miracle worker.

That's not an ideal state to have a baby.

And the person has to be there mentally and emotionally, too, saying, "I'm ready to make these changes."

Because having a child is a huge change, so they have to kind of be in that spot where they can put their own selfish life behind.

There are different stages that women go through, and they say that the first one is the maiden where it's all about you.

You're in school, you're doing your thing, like a lot of women go through in their early 20s, and it's all about me.

And once they become the mother stage, it's self-sacrificing. It doesn't necessarily have to be a baby.

For me, it's my business, this is my baby right now.

You have to give up a lot and sacrifice things for that, and then you get to menopause age, you're the crone or this wise woman.

So, there's the three different stages that women go through in their lives, and I thought it was very fascinating that they each have a purpose.

Kim: So, could make these lifestyle changes congruently with acupuncture and Chinese medicine and still have success?

Let's say you did them together, really started exercising, eating better, reduced your stress, came in here and did the acupuncture and Chinese herbs for, let's say three to six months, like you mentioned, but at the same time.

Could you potentially see the same results, or would you recommend starting a little bit sooner before coming to do additional therapy?

Stephanie: I mean, it's always going to be better to have a longer length of time with a better lifestyle, but a lot of patients come in, they just don't know what to do.

They don't know if they're doing the right thing or the wrong thing or anything really.

So yeah, when they make those changes, for some people, it's very quick. The quickest patient I had was about 3 weeks.

She was on medication for her allergies that was drying up cervical mucus and the doctor never told her that it could affect her fertility.

She got off of it, and then we did acupuncture and herbs to help her with her sinuses along with her fertility, and she was pregnant in 3 weeks, but of course that's not the typical.

Stephanie: A lot of women come in and they don't know why they're not getting pregnant, and they don't have the answers because the doctors don't always do all of these tests.

You know, like with endometriosis, they're not going to do that first thing, and then they go, "Oh, well this is a problem."

But we can tell with a pulse, "Okay, there's a blood flow issue here."

Whether it's cysts or whatever, let's say you don't even have that diagnosis, we can figure out what the underlying issue is that would cause that, and we're treating that.

So that's really important for you to actually understand the why because a lot of doctors don't tell you.

They're just like, "Well, you have this. It's bad luck, or a bad omen," or something, you know?

In Chinese medicine, we say, "Okay, why do they have that?"

And with most doctors, you ask them a why, they get mad at you or they just blow you off, they probably won't really give you any explanation because they likely don't really know.

And that's really important for patients to know, something going on.

And it might be something very small, it might be something big, it might be various things, but at least they know, and then they can work on it.

Kim: So, for me, for instance, I have possible PCOS, never really formally diagnosed, definitely endometriosis, definitely diagnosed.

I guess I've never really asked why.

So, can you tell me the "why" for my specific issues?

Stephanie: We call it blood stagnation in Chinese medicine.

It's basically where blood is kind of like sludgy, and thick, and not moving, and stuck.

So, we do herbs that are going to improve blood flow, open up, dilate the blood vessels.

For a lot of people it's lifestyle and diet changes and things like that which over time can cause a lot of poor circulation and stagnation.

Kim: So conceivably, if everything starts moving and going the way that it should be, then you should see visible changes during menstruation, I imagine, then?

For instance, less clotting.

Stephanie: Exactly, because obviously there's pregnancy and there's non-pregnancy, but there's so many things in between that.

So, how do we know if you're improving in your fertility besides the pregnancy?

It would be that your periods are more regular, you're not having clotting, you're not cramping, you're not getting crazy mood swings, things like that.

But obviously, for the IVF patients, we have to throw that out because the medications are going to do irritate these things that we can't control because basically what they do is they shut down the body, they shut down the pituitary so it can't secrete hormones, and then they give you the hormones to do it on its own.

So, it's totally controlled by those medications so that they can time everything exactly right, because otherwise, it's kind of a little bit of a guessing game.

But what's great when combining IVF and acupuncture is that we can greatly reduce the side effects, so the cramping, the bloating, the mood swings, irritability, all those things that can be caused from the medications.

We can also treat Ovarian Hyper Stimulation Syndrome.

Kim: I know myself and many friends speak so highly of Chinese Medicine, so thank you so much for taking this time with me and sharing your thoughts.

Stephanie: You're welcome.

Here are Stephanie's impressive list of credentials:

- Nationally licensed Doctor of Oriental Medicine & Licensed Acupuncture Physician (NCCAOM)
- Certified Functional Medicine Practitioner (CFMP)
- NCCAOM certified Chinese Herbalist
- Functional Medicine University graduate
- Doctoral Program, Pacific College of Oriental Medicine
- Master's Degree in Oriental Medicine, Summa cum laude – Florida College of Integrative Medicine
- Bachelor's Degree in Professional Health Studies – Florida College of Integrative Medicine
- Associate of Science Degree in Medical Massage Therapy

Her certifications and specialties include:

- Certified Functional Medicine Practitioner (CFMP) – Functional Medicine University
- Featured guest and panel member on Chinese Medicine That Works Blog Talk Radio

- Panel member on Practical Chinese Herbology
- Featured Chinese Medicine Expert – Fox 35 News
- Advanced Certification in Contemporary Chinese Pulse Diagnosis – Dr. Leon Hammer, MD
- Associate Instructor of Contemporary Chinese Pulse Diagnosis
- Published author – Chinese Medicine Quarterly & Velocity Magazine
- Certified Facial Enhance Practitioner – Paul Adkins

Chapter 12: A Success Story

"Sometimes in tragedy we find out life's purpose the eye sheds a tear to find its focus." – Robert Brault

I sat down and asked a few fertility patients to share their experiences and recommendations to others just starting their journey.

They shared their thoughts on the process and the things they wished they'd known earlier.

I first sat down with my friend Kirsten, 37, who has been trying to conceive for 2 ½ years.

After having tried to conceive for 1 year, they were finally successful.

They were so excited and filled with anticipation for their first ultrasound appointment at 8 weeks.

Heartbreak quickly ensued as they were informed that there was no heartbeat.

Following their miscarriage, they tried to conceive again on their own for another 6 months.

When they weren't able to get pregnant again, they decided it was time to go to a fertility doctor.

It was then that Kirsten was diagnosed with ovulatory disfunction.

For the next year and a half, they went through 3 months of Clomid, 3 timed cycles with ovulation induction, and 3 IVF egg retrievals.

She had always lead a healthy lifestyle, but before her 3rd egg retrieval, she decided it was time to make some serious changes.

She started eating even better, stopped drinking alcohol, did acupuncture and took more vitamins than anyone should on a daily basis.

Her 3rd retrieval was a huge success!

The first 2 yielded no normal embryos and the 3rd resulted in 3 PGS tested, normal embryos and 1 mosaic embryo.

This was such a massive improvement over the other 2 retrievals and such a shock to both her and her husband.

She continued these healthy habits and shortly after, they transferred an embryo which resulted in a healthy pregnancy!

Here is what Kirsten had to share:

Telling people the truth is easier than keeping IVF or any fertility treatments a secret.

It takes so much more effort to make up an excuse for why you're turning down a cocktail at a wedding instead of just saying you're currently going through an IVF cycle.

Or lying about why you're rushing off from dinner early so you can give yourself an injection.

Or inventing a reason for why you can't make a trip out of town with friends because you have to plan around specifically-timed IVF procedures.

Or making up reasons for all the times you have to come into the office late or leave early for appointments at the fertility clinic.

Or having to pretend you're happy around friends when you're crushed because you just got dealt bad news about egg retrieval, your embryo results, etc.

When I decided to be honest with people around me about it, it was one less thing to worry about in a process where there's so much to worry about.

And it's how you start to learn that many people around may know someone or be going through the infertility struggle themselves.

Infertility is a painful, anxiety-ridden experience for a couple.

It tries you emotionally, financially, and rules your entire life for an undetermined amount of time.

You don't get any guidance on how to navigate, cope, and support each other through the process.

But while the experience is brutal, my husband and I did eventually grow closer, and our marriage stronger, in spite of it.

I had a handful of friends and family members with whom I shared more specific details about my IVF procedures with frequently check in with me after key appointments, procedures, PGS tests, etc.

I appreciated that because sometimes I felt self-conscious bringing up the topic on my own because I worried whether people cared to hear about every nitty gritty detail.

So, when loved ones remembered to text me after an appointment to ask how things went or during injections to ask how I was hanging in there, it meant a lot to me because it made me feel like they were emotionally invested in my IVF experience too.

And it was an open invitation to talk about it without me feeling like I was forcing the topic on them.

So much hurrying followed by so much waiting.

There are stages of IVF that are a chaotic scramble requiring daily injections, back-to-back doctor's appointments, blood test, ultrasounds, and procedures scheduled from one day to the next.

And then after, you sit and wait for rounds and rounds of various results for days and weeks- how many embryos made it to day 5, how many tested genetically normal, did my embryo implant successfully, will I get a positive pregnancy test, will there be a heartbeat seen at my six-week ultrasound?

You have no choice but to let go of control during fertility treatments.

Trying to plan for when your fertility treatments can begin and how long they will take, how many rounds will be required before you succeed, and how to respond when things don't go according to plan is impossible.

If you can accept the idea that your body is not a machine, and it won't respond the same way to treatments from one cycle to the next or the way another woman responds, it will make it easier to cope.

Focus on what you can control to help you stay sane - taking your supplements, eating well, eliminating toxins, exercising, yoga and acupuncture, seeking support when you need it, and consulting with your doctor about the nagging questions in the back of your mind.

Also letting go of how you imagined you would build your family so you can be open to other ways of having children if fertility treatments fail.

Once I started to consider options like donor egg, adoption, it gave me a new sense of hope because it didn't feel like our last door to parenthood was about to close if IVF failed again.

Last but not least, cost savings.

Insurance providers are all over the board about fertility treatment coverage, especially in states that don't mandate coverage.

Be an FBI investigator when it comes to understanding pricing for fertility medications and treatment.

Ask questions from financial counselors at fertility clinics.

Learn what makes sense to pay out of pocket versus letting insurance providers pick up the tab.

For example, fertility medications are still less expensive if you self-pay than having to pay fertility procedures like egg retrievals and embryo transfers out of pocket.

Use pharmacies that offer special discounts to self-pay patients.

Ask about discount pricing packages available for fertility treatments if you're self-paying.

Made in the USA
Coppell, TX
28 January 2021

48983810R00127